Advance Praise

'Emma Fogarty is a truly exceptional person. Her bravery and positive outlook in the face of enormous challenges are monumental. Her life story is one of constant pain, enduring love and resilience beyond comprehension.'

Ray D'Arcy

'This is not just a story of pain – it's a story of power, bravery, perseverance, resilience and the beauty of the human spirit. Emma's journey is raw, real and deeply inspiring. I'm honoured to walk through life with her as my friend.'

Trisha Lewis, *Trisha's Transformation*

'I met Emma for the first time about fifteen years ago. I hadn't heard about EB until that day. Since then, I have been an ambassador for Debra Ireland. Watching the pain that EB patients go through is heartbreaking. Emma has displayed courage and bravery which has been an inspiration to me during my career but also in my life. We have stayed in contact over the years and tried to raise awareness of EB as much as we can. This book encapsulates what people with EB go through every day and also what their families go through every day. Emma is the oldest living patient with EB, so for her to put down on paper what she goes through must have been tough, but she is tough.'

Johnny Sexton

Emma Fogarty is a writer, activist and advocate living with epidermolysis bullosa (EB), a rare and painful skin condition. At forty-one in 2025, she is the oldest living Irish person with her form of the condition, continuing to defy the odds with her extraordinary strength and resilience, as well as her remarkable achievements, including taking part in the 2024 Dublin Marathon.

Being Emma

Living My Best Life with Butterfly Skin

EMMA FOGARTY

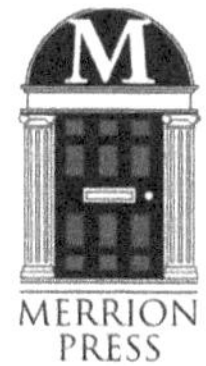

First published in 2025 by
Merrion Press
10 George's Street
Newbridge
Co. Kildare
Ireland
www.merrionpress.ie

978 1 78537 568 2 (Paper)
978 1 78537 574 3 (eBook)

A CIP catalogue record for this book is available from the British Library.

Typeset in Sabon LT Pro and Binter Display

Cover design by riverdesignbooks.com

Front cover image © Richard Sheehy
www.richardsheehyphotography.com

Butterfly vector © daphnedesign/Shutterstock

Merrion Press is a member of Publishing Ireland.

To my mother and father,
for taking me home.

Contents

Author's Note

Some of the names in this book have been changed to protect the identity of those involved in certain incidents.

Foreword

Colin Farrell

My friend Emma Fogarty is truly one of the most extraordinary women I have ever had the good fortune of meeting. We've been friends for some fifteen years now, and since our first meeting our friendship and knowledge of each other's lives has deepened, as tends to happen over time. I feel in a very fortunate position to be at the receiving end of her kindness and generosity, her spirited humour and sense of fun.

I also feel uncommonly blessed that she pulls no punches in her sharing of life's struggles, the totality of her story. Emma has always been keen never to feel sorry for herself. She is quick to remind me and others that there is always someone worse off. And yet, the constant and excruciating pain she lives with, by being trapped in a body that has been punishing to inhabit, is real.

Her journey in and through life has been a remarkable one. Born with a cruel and debilitating disease, whose sole concern is to inflict pain and suffering upon those who live with it, she has defied the odds in so many ways. It's indeed a miracle that she is still with us, and our lives – everyone fortunate enough to encounter her – have become more rich for that fact. But Emma's greatest defiance is not that she has lived to see her forty-first birthday, though doctors – as soon as she was born – said she would live only weeks. Her greatest defiance is her insistence on living a full and meaningful life. A life of adventure and joy. A life that is, of course, limited in many ways by epidermolysis bullosa, but a life that has shared so much laughter, so much friendship, had so many challenges chosen and imposed, and has triumphed over them all.

It is not that Emma is still alive that is the miracle. It is how Emma has chosen to live in the face of such adversity that is the true miracle. Her story is one that I feel needs to be shared. I have, in our years as friends, derived incredible hope through the power of her spirit. I have also felt anger and pain at what she has had to go through. And … I have been baffled by her courage. She squirms when I say such things, but it's just the way it is.

I'm so thrilled she has decided to share her story. It is a story not only of an individual's call to arms in the daily fight of having a warrior spirit trapped in a battle-broken body. It is also a family story. Of her mother, Pat, and father, Malachy, and her sister, Catherine. The love they have shared. The triumph of that love through all the challenges life has thrown in their shared path.

Emma's life is an extraordinary one and she is quite simply a beautiful and powerful human being. She's one of the greatest teachers we have, and if the reader can feel even an ounce of the wonder, the sorrow, the strength and hope that I have felt in knowing her, then they will walk away with a life enriched for the time spent in the company of this amazing woman.

Los Angeles
June 2025

What Is Butterfly Skin?

Epidermolysis bullosa (EB), commonly nicknamed 'butterfly skin', is a rare genetic condition that makes a person's skin incredibly fragile – so fragile that even small things most people wouldn't notice, like rubbing against bedsheets or wearing shoes, can cause painful blisters or open wounds. People with EB are often called 'butterfly children' because their skin is as delicate as a butterfly's wing.

On the surface, skin with EB may look normal. But underneath, the layers don't hold together the way they should. So the skin can peel apart simply from friction – walking, hugging, eating, even sleeping. For some, the condition is relatively mild. For others, it affects not only the skin but also the eyes, mouth, throat and internal linings of the body.

In the most severe forms, it can be life-threatening.

EB is caused by a fault in the genes that means the proteins needed to hold the skin together are missing. These are like the glue or anchors that keep the skin's structure in place. If the gene is damaged or missing, the body can't make those anchors properly. Which gene is affected determines what type of EB someone has. Some people inherit it from one parent, others from both. In most cases, it's something a person is born with and lives with every day of their life.

One of the more serious forms of EB is called Recessive Dystrophic EB. In this type, the faulty gene affects collagen –

specifically collagen type VII, a protein that normally forms tiny rope-like structures called anchoring fibrils. These fibrils work like nails, holding the top layer of skin to the layer beneath it. Without them, the skin slides and tears easily, often leaving deep wounds that scar. Over time, the constant damage can cause the fingers and toes to fuse, and even simple acts like eating or swallowing can become incredibly painful and even impossible if the lining of the throat is affected.

People with EB also suffer from osteoporosis. This can make life even harder and more painful, suffering constant breaks and bone disintegration.

Living with EB means daily bandaging, constant wound care and a lifetime of managing pain, risk of infection and complications.

There is no cure.

Prologue

I'm a Survivor

My mother tells me that when I was born the room fell deathly silent. She knew something was wrong, but she didn't know what. Neither did the nurses, nor the doctor they rushed to find.

That silence didn't last because I began to cry, and my mother tells me I didn't stop at all. Because I was born in terrible pain.

My name is Emma Fogarty and I've just turned forty-one. I live in Abbeyleix, in a nice home with views of the fields, and I love my fashion, my shoes, my music and a glass of bubbly at any opportunity.

Oh, and I have a genetic skin condition called epidermolysis bullosa. We shorten that mouthful to EB. What it means is that I'm missing the collagen that sits between the layers of my skin. I'll explain it to you this way. Imagine that your skin is attached to your muscle with a sort of Velcro. Well, I don't have the Velcro at all and so there's nothing giving my skin any stick. The layers of my skin just float around on top of each other. Skin is fragile anyway, but with no collagen, if I get hit, my skin tears like paper.

And there is nothing anyone can do about it.

With my form of EB, both parents have to have a faulty gene to cause the condition. Of course, my parents didn't know that when their eyes met across a dance hall in Limerick, and they didn't know it when they married and when my mom was pregnant with me. The first time they knew of it was when they were told what was wrong with their new baby. And it was a while before they heard the words 'epidermolysis bullosa' at all. The first thing said to them by the doctor was that I would not live a week.

Maybe the fact that I did survive the week, and the next one, and the year, and on and on, formed in me a sort of stubborn insistence that I would live and I would be happy. Because I am. I love my life and I love living every day of it, even the hardest ones. And there are plenty of those.

You see, I have EB, but it is not *me*; EB is not who I *am*. EB is a condition I *have*. But I am not my skin. I am Emma. I am Catherine's sister, Pat and Malachy's daughter, Kim's friend. I've got a life behind me and a life ahead of me. Just like you.

This is my story.

Part One

Becoming Emma

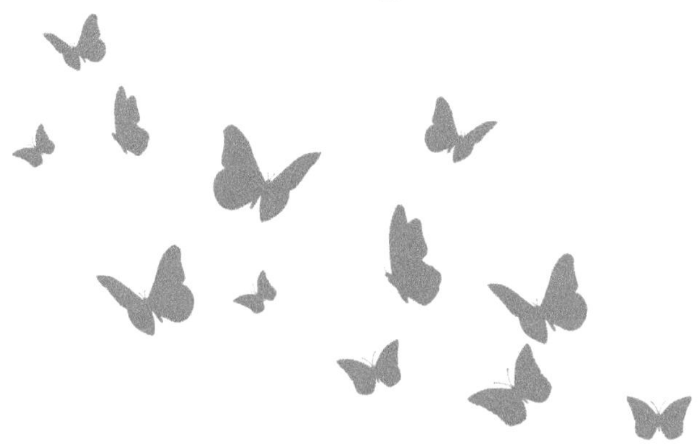

1

Delicate

You probably haven't heard of EB. Most people haven't. It's not something that gets big news coverage or massive awareness campaigns. There aren't films about it.

But for the people who live with it – and for their families – it's our whole lives.

Epidermolysis bullosa doesn't exactly roll off the tongue – it sounds like something scientific you read about in journals, but that's not what it's like when you have it.

In real life, EB is up close and personal.

Imagine your skin is as fragile as paper. Imagine a hug can cause a wound. Imagine that wearing clothes can tear your skin. EB makes the simple things brutal.

There's no cure, not yet, though researchers always promise them. There's not even a treatment, not in the way most people would think of it. With EB it's all about management. Daily, long, painful routines just to keep the body safe and us sufferers alive.

For me, with the type of EB I have, it's a full-time job. For me, EB means bandage changes every second day that take up to four hours, and partial changes in between. It means infections that need constant monitoring, skin that won't heal properly and pain that no painkiller ever quite covers. EB, for me, means being always cautious, always careful, yet still, somehow, always covered in wounds.

Some people's bodies carry them through the world. My body has always needed a *plan*, always needed someone else to help.

And so, I have never experienced freedom.

But ...

EB is not my whole story. It's a part of me. A big part, yes, but not the only part.

Because EB has given me a viewpoint I don't think I would have had otherwise. It has made me see the world differently. It has taught me patience, resilience, compassion. It has taught me how to listen – really listen – to other people's pain. And it has made me stubborn in the best way – EB has made me really determined.

EB has also given me community. Through Debra Ireland, through other families and kids like me, I've found people who *get it*. People who don't need it explained. That's a rare gift and a precious one.

People always ask, 'Is EB rare?' and the answer is yes – it's very rare. Fewer than 300 people in Ireland have it. However, just because it's rare doesn't mean it's not worth talking about. It's the rare things that need shouting about the most. Because when you're rare, sometimes you're at risk of being forgotten.

People also ask me, 'Do you wish you didn't have EB?' and that's a complicated one. Of course I do. Of course I wish I could run, or wear what I like, or stand at a concert for hours without pain. But I also know that EB shaped me – my values, my choices, my voice. EB made me who I am. And I like who I am.

So yeah, EB is brutal. It's exhausting. It's unforgiving. But I am still here.

That's EB. And that's me.

* * *

When my mother, Pat, was pregnant with me, there was no need for anyone to worry. It was her first baby and things went along as normal. There were no warning signs, no unusual scans. Labour went ahead with no alarm bells, nothing to cause any concern.

But as soon as I arrived into the world, all of our lives – my mother's, my father's and mine – were changed. I was born badly wounded, with no skin at all on my arm or left foot, and they didn't know why. Then a nurse tried to feed me and the metal edge of her little nurse's watch hit off my cheek and pulled the skin off it. Just a normal smooth-sided watch – something every nurse used to wear – and it injured me so badly. My skin was like tissue paper.

'We don't know what's wrong with this baby,' the doctor said to my mom and dad and, just like that, the floor dropped out from under them.

The doctors were baffled. They sent a sample of my skin away for testing. As they waited, my parents rang their loved ones. My dad's mother, Nana Fogarty, set down the phone and made arrangements to get up to Dublin. As soon as she could, she drove to the hospital without stopping. I imagine she prayed all the way there.

By the time Nana Fogarty arrived in the hospital, I had been baptised, just in case. In those days, Ireland was still fully immersed in the idea that purgatory and limbo existed, and so, within hours of my birth, a priest was called. He blessed some tap water and gently poured it over my head. That was my christening. Just Mom, Dad and the priest were there. My name, chosen quickly from the shortlist they'd hoped to mull over, was Emma.

Also by the time Nana Fogarty got there, the biopsy results had come back. My parents had an answer. Now they knew what was wrong with this baby.

The words were new to everyone in the room: epidermolysis bullosa. The words that would come to define my whole life.

'She won't live a week,' the paediatrician said. And just like that, my life was given an expiry date. Just like that, there was a ticking clock.

He added something else. 'I'm sorry to say this, but she would be better off if she didn't.'

* * *

My aunt Angela was the first person my mom told.

'Her skin is like paper,' she said, 'I don't know what to do.'

Angela hung up the phone and ran straight away across the back fields behind her house to bang on the door of a nurse she knew. She wouldn't have known this woman well enough to bang on her door like that, but she did it anyway because she just needed something, *anything* – an answer that would give my mother hope.

The nurse told her everything she knew, but her words hurt. 'Babies with that condition rarely make it,' she said, 'and if they do it's a very hard illness to live with; there will be no quality of life whatsoever.'

I've been told this story so many times it plays in my

head like a film – my aunt running all that way to get hope, information, a reason. I don't know what it would have felt like for my family to hear such devastating news delivered so sharply. Although I definitely know what that baby would have felt when her skin tore. Because I still feel that every day and have done for my entire life.

I couldn't suck on a bottle because the rubber tore my lips, so I was a ball of frustration until they figured out how to drip milk into my mouth. My mother cut a hole in the teat so the milk could be brought out without much work, and I was fed that way – drop by drop, hour by hour.

On my mom's side, the Bowens mobilised and gathered in Angela's house – my aunts Marguerite, Martina, Marie and my uncle Sean – to start making baby clothes inside out so the seams wouldn't harm me. They sewed through the night to get clothes to Mom so she could dress me.

That memory, though it's not mine directly, burns so vividly in my heart.

Aunt Angela, God bless her, also bought me my first doll. I still have it, a little soft thing with long legs and closed eyes stitched on. Sleeping Dolly became her name. I clung to her then and sometimes still cling to her now. Sleeping Dolly became one of those sacred belongings that babies (and grown-ups) cannot be without. Myself and Sleeping Dolly have been through a lot.

* * *

I spent the first few months of my life in Crumlin Hospital, in and out of incubators.

Despite what the doctor had said, I lived a week, then a

month, and when I was three months old, my parents asked if they could take me home.

'We are sorry for you,' came the reply, 'but your child will not live for long.'

'I think Emma is a survivor,' my mother said.

'Well, if she lives,' came the reply, 'she will have a very hard life. You can take her home.'

So they did. They brought me home to where we still live today, in Abbeyleix.

That was probably the moment when my parents could have given up on me. No one would have blamed them. They'd been told I could never survive this condition. But I think my mother decided then and there that even if that *was* the case, I *would* have a life. Not an existence, a *life*. Even if it was just a few months or a year, there would be family and friends and adventures.

* * *

When my parents left the hospital with me in their arms, Aunt Angela showed up with a camera and started snapping photos.

Mom turned to her and told her to stop.

'I won't,' Angela said. 'Emma wasn't supposed to live a week and look at her now, coming home.' For her it was a momentous day.

She took a whole roll of film of me that day. I'm glad she did because I have the photos now and I will admit I was a *very* cute little baby.

Then, one day not long after I came home, Nana Fogarty rang and told my parents she had found another Irish family whose little boy had EB too. That felt like a light shining through the dark for my parents, and they went to visit them the very next time they were in Limerick – coincidentally, my parents are both from there and this child came from nearby.

'This is Bobby,' his parents said as soon as they opened the door. My parents looked down at a little boy with blistered skin. He was playing with his toys, happy out, on the floor of the sitting room.

Just seeing Bobby there so happy gave my parents real hope. It also gave them something else: a connection to another family who knew exactly what they were going through. This family were ahead on the road they were just starting out on, and they gave my parents the promise that I could make it along that road too.

My parents could have wrapped me up in cotton wool and kept me in a box – I was small enough. But on that day they decided they wouldn't. Their daughter wasn't going to spend her life in the shadow of EB. No matter how long I lived, I would be out in the open.

If this family and this boy could do it, so could we.

My parents were open-minded in ways that you don't always see in people who find themselves faced with something so brutal. They refused to see me as broken. It was never what can't Emma do? It was always what *can* Emma do?

That's something I carried into every year that followed and maybe it's where I get my stubborn streak and determination.

I wasn't supposed to make it to my first birthday, but I did.

I wasn't supposed to go to school. But I did.

I wasn't supposed to see my tens, my twenties, my thirties, my forties.

But I *did.*

There is a power in being underestimated – is that the lesson we take from this? Maybe those words – 'she won't live a week' – went in. Even as a newborn, did I hear those words somehow and did they make me brave?

I had nothing to lose by being scrappy. The world goes around regardless, whether you're here or not, so you may as well cling on. And maybe because of the start I had, the pain I felt from the beginning, it gave me a sense that even when you fall, even when it hurts so much your eyes water and your chest heaves, you just *have* to keep going.

Because it's worth it. It's so worth it to be alive.

My parents didn't give up on me, they didn't hand me back to the hospital and say this is too difficult. They didn't shrink from the hard work of keeping me alive. They rolled up their sleeves, got on with it and taught me to do the same.

And that's what I've done every day since.

2

Try

To my family I was simply a normal child who needed extra care. I didn't know what it was to have normal skin. For me, it was a case of realising as soon as I learned to walk that falling meant real pain.

My mother was on the phone to the doctor when she first saw me stand up, hands out in front of me, starting to toddle across the room in front of her. She told the doctor she had to go, not so she could get the camera, but because she needed to make sure I didn't fall. And after the first few times, I learned falling was not something I could easily recover from. So I avoided it as much as I could.

I was a little girl who walked and didn't run, who took care when getting up or down from the couch or my mom's lap. I was never going to do tumbles, but I wasn't upset by that. I didn't want to do those things because I knew the consequences. I knew the risk wasn't worth the reward, not for me. I was absolutely content sitting on the floor playing with my little dolls and my teddies.

Still, my memories of being little are just like yours: playing in the garden or my bedroom, watching TV, going on outings with cousins. Sitting in the back of the family car on the way down to my Nana Fogarty's, looking out the window every time my mom said, 'Horses, Emma, look!'

Dad taught in secondary school, maths and geography, but he could cover a bit of everything when needed. He started off in a small school in Abbeyleix, and later, when the population of Laois grew a bit, his little school got absorbed into the larger community school. That's where he stayed until he retired.

I remember one year when I was really small, maybe only three, the school Dad taught at was putting on a show, *Oliver Twist*, and they were stuck for the role of Fagin. Totally against character, Dad said he would do it. I don't know how reluctantly, but I do know he learned the songs, the lines, the whole thing, and he sang them over and over at home until *we* knew them too.

When the night of the play came, Mom and I went along to the school to see it. I was excited, waiting for my dad to come on. Anyway, the lights dimmed, the music started and on came this man – this scraggly, bearded old rogue of a character.

Mom leaned down and whispered, 'There's Daddy.'

Well, I wasn't having a bar of that. *That* wasn't my dad, that was some stranger with a beard dancing around the stage. And when Dad came down after the show, still in costume, and tried to sit beside us and coax me onto his lap, I refused point blank. No matter how much my mom tried to convince me it was Daddy, I would not believe it. In my child's mind I thought Dad could only ever look one way. He had to take the beard off before I would so much as consider that it was him at all. Then I got it. It's a cute memory.

Even though I cried a lot, I was a happy child. My parents took me to Lourdes when I was six, just after I started school. I don't remember much about it, but I know we stayed in a hotel. One thing I do remember is the nuns dipping me in and out of the cold baths and my mother warning them, 'Gently! Gently!' –

of course they weren't gentle and so I screamed the whole time. But in the evening people gathered together and sang lovely folk songs. I thought that was great craic. I would sit on whichever knee would have me and enjoy the music.

I started Junior Infants in Scoil Mhuire in Abbeyleix at five. I knew most of the kids in my class already – we'd been together in play school. Abbeyleix is the kind of small town where everyone knew who you were – especially if you were me.

The teachers knew us too. They knew who might need help with reading, who might cry if their mam was late, and who (me) needed to be handled with a little more care. Not that they ever made a big show of it. They were just kind. And I loved it there.

I didn't think it was special that I was going to school, but the local paper did. They took my picture and wrote a whole article describing me as a miracle child who was going to school. I didn't get it at all, not at six. I could hardly see *myself* as a miracle. I still don't. I have always seen myself as just Emma. But, of course, it was a miracle. All the odds were stacked against me.

For me, going to school was an obvious step. *Now* I know that my parents were behind the scenes, working with the school and speaking to the other parents, asking them to explain to their children that they needed to be gentle with Emma and why. And so, of course, on my first day I was something of interest. But kids don't tend to dwell on things, and before long I was just Emma to them too.

I loved primary school because of that. I didn't get stared at. I wasn't different or unusual. I was simply a classmate, the one who came in after everyone else was sitting down and the one who left just before the bell rang, to avoid getting jostled in the crowd.

My mother drove me to school at first, as slowly as she could without causing a traffic jam, taking the bumps in the road at five miles an hour. Ours was a busy school and cars would pull up outside and let the children out, and so would she – though a bit later than everyone else – and I would walk inside like every other child.

I loved that small moment of being by myself, because I was rarely ever by myself.

* * *

My first few years of school were mostly just like yours, with tadpoles and *márla* and learning the letters phonetically in songs, only I couldn't do PE and I couldn't go out to the yard. I would observe other children as I walked along, watching for the smallest sign that they might move unexpectedly – the lowering of a shoulder, the twitch of a hand. If there was a group of children ahead of me, I would give them a wide berth and hope to get by before someone started a sudden game of chase. I still do that.

The teacher would ask for volunteers, usually four, to stay inside with me at lunch time and play in the classroom. There was something about that – access to the classroom without a teacher – that made every hand in the class go up. That became my thing. Staying in at lunch with eager volunteers.

As well as my first day at school, another milestone was my First Communion, where the whole family got together and dressed for the occasion. I had the little white dress, little soft ballet slippers and a silk halo on my head with ribbons down the back. I even wore gloves, and I was delighted with myself. I still have the little white drawstring bag that you see on the arms of little girls all over Ireland on that special day.

Afterwards, we had people back to our house for a cup of tea and I was slipped pound notes and fivers, which I stuffed into that little bag. I'd imagine I put it in the post office, and it might still be there because I don't remember ever taking it out!

* * *

As I got older, I took the chance of going out to the yard at school a few times. It was too enticing, hearing the big games planned. I'd convince myself I could play too, convince myself I could avoid a bump. I never could, not with one group playing football and another playing chase. Once I turned just in time to see a football heading straight for me.

'You gave it a header, Emma!' the lads kept shouting over in good spirits, but I could see they were worried.

I was okay. No skin tore, but I did have to go home. I soon learned that going out was never worth it.

3

The Lucky One

There were some things I pushed for. Things I was told 'maybe not' or 'be careful' about. And most of the time, I didn't ask again, out of sense. But there were certain things that just got stuck in my head and wouldn't shift.

I wanted a bicycle.

The crusade for a bike started, as many things did, from a window. I would sit watching from the back of Mom's car, on the way to school, as kids – my classmates and neighbours – flew past on their bikes with their hair wild and their coats flapping. They had freedom written all over their faces – and I wanted it.

Mom and Dad tried to turn me off. Soft suggestions at first, then firmer. 'Maybe wait a bit, pet,' they'd say. 'It's not safe.' But I was stubborn.

I *wanted* a bicycle.

In the end, Santa brought me a bike. When I woke up on Christmas morning, there it was, blue and pink, parked under the tree like a dream come true. It had two stabilisers on the back and tassels on the handles. I looked at it with a mix of joy and fear. It was everything I had wanted, but this was real now, and real meant risk.

I couldn't just imagine it any more. I had to actually get on it and go.

The first time, my mom held the back of the seat as I climbed on. I could barely breathe from the nerves.

'Mom,' I said, 'I really want to ride the bike. But I'm so afraid of falling.'

She said, 'Emma, pet, I'll hold on as long as I can.'

And she did. She walked holding tight to the back of the seat while I pedalled along shakily, and I remember saying over and over, 'Don't let go, Mom, don't.'

When we reached the end of the path, she squatted down, looked me in the eye, and said, 'Emma, I have to let go now or you'll never do it.'

So we made a deal. She let go and I learned to pedal by myself.

My bike became one of my most treasured possessions. Sometimes I'd even cycle to school, my mother trailing behind me on foot with her heart in her mouth. The road had a slight downhill slope, which made it easy for my little legs. Mom would wheel the bike home and collect me in the car later – I'd never have made it back up the hill. But that arrangement still gave me the independence I wanted so much.

There's a photo of me on that bike. If you saw it, you'd think nothing of it. Just a little girl about to cycle down the road, hair in a bob, her hands gripping the handlebars. A girl child on a bicycle is ordinary, it's normal.

That's what I love most about my memories of my childhood. Because that's how it felt. It was *my* normal, *my* girlhood.

Just Emma. Me.

Looking back, I realise how intentional it all was. Everyone around me was trying their best to build me some semblance of normality in an extraordinary situation. Because of that, I could live in the real world, where kids get bikes for Christmas.

The adults around me built that place, where safety didn't mean saying no to everything. It was more about finding ways to say yes.

And look, of course I fell off my bike. Poor Mom had to pick me up screaming off the ground more than once. On one occasion I was riding in circles around the house, faster and faster, when the wheel clipped the edge of a step and down I went.

Mom heard me scream before I even realised I had hit the ground, and she was there in seconds, scooping me up. My hands, knees, feet were raw. There was blood everywhere. I was screaming, overwhelmed by the horrible, hot stinging and throbbing that EB patients know too well.

'I just want my cat,' I said, delirious as she carried me in to the sofa.

'Get her the cat,' my mom said to my dad over her shoulder as she laid me down there. Dad hesitated because, of course, I had wounds and there was the risk of infection.

As my wails got louder, my mom said, 'For God's sake, Malachy, get the cat!'

God love him, my dad went outside and searched high and low for the cat. I don't know how long it took him to find her, but eventually he brought her in to me – a reluctant nurse.

I got back on that bike. The feeling of independence was too beautiful to let go of because of one bad fall. But eventually I outgrew it and, with it, the possibility of riding a bike ever again. Back in the 1990s in rural Ireland they didn't stock stabilisers for bigger bikes. There was no Amazon, no eBay. In those days whatever the local shop stocked was what you could work with, and if it didn't have what you needed, well, tough.

It wasn't fair, but it wasn't anyone's fault. It was just one of the freedoms you have to let go of as a person with different needs.

I think that's why, even now, when I see products being made that could have helped me – large trikes or adapted bikes, clothes without seams – I feel warm and hopeful. It's great to see these things because it means little children with EB can have childhoods that are 'normal'. It feels like the world is finally catching up.

* * *

There was in Ireland in the 1990s a small community of people with EB. It is such a rare disorder by any measure, but for those living with it, there is a huge need for medical care. So our dermatologist, Dr Rosemarie Watson, created a monthly clinic where all the clinicians we needed to see would have the same space on the same day so we could see them all at once, and they could see us – all the children in Ireland with butterfly skin, all ages, all gathered in the same place.

It was a smart idea and it really worked. The experts could coordinate with each other and pass files back and forth. It was also a godsend for our parents. They could swap stories, tips and, of course, sorrows. Most of all it was great for us, the kids. It meant less stress, fewer journeys to the hospital, and we also had the benefit of seeing others who looked like us and moved like us. We weren't alone. There were other children who were in pain like us. In a world where most people didn't even know EB existed, that meant something.

The waiting room was the usual – rows of hard chairs, walls covered in information and a smorgasbord of random magazines. Why is it always *Woman's Way* and *National Geographic*? There were some toys there too, but most of us couldn't play with them. We didn't mind. We'd sit beside each other and play our own games that didn't involve getting down on the floor.

Years later, Dr Watson told me something I'll never forget.

'You know, Emma,' she said, 'I saw you in the paediatrics corridor one day, waiting to be seen. And I thought, *This little girl needs her own specialised care.*'

Dr Watson did it all herself. She went from there and learned everything there was to learn about EB. She trained in EB care and had her nurses do the same. She built the clinic around that one moment in a corridor. Around *me*.

Imagine that.

One child, one day, and Dr Watson changed everything, for all of us. She became my doctor for nearly thirty years. She still sits on the board of Debra Ireland. She has guided many, many families through the storm that my parents went through alone.

When Dr Watson told me that story, I didn't feel overwhelmed. Not exactly. I felt a kind of weight, but not a bad one, and definitely not a burden. Just the weight of awareness that something in me and my life had sparked a chain reaction that made things better for other people. What do you even do with that?

Why was it me she saw and not someone else? Why did she choose that moment to act? I don't have the answers, but I've always felt, deep down, that I was meant to help others. I've always felt there was something in me that needed to be shared.

That story made me think about purpose. Maybe it's my will to live – not just exist, but *live*. Maybe it's my stubborn refusal to be shut away from the world. Or maybe I was just the right person at the right time.

Whatever it was, I'm grateful. And I'm proud.

Crumlin Hospital has always been such a huge part of my life. It was my first home; I was taken there straight from Kilkenny where I was born.

I remember once walking down one of the corridors, when a nurse stopped me and said, 'Emma? Emma Fogarty?'

I didn't know this nurse. How did she know me? It turned out she was the first nurse to hold me in Crumlin. She told me how proud she was of me.

We talked and laughed and hugged each other in that corridor. I never got her name. I was still just a teenager and I didn't think to ask. But I wish I had.

***

Our little clinic and that waiting room full of families eventually led to something bigger – Debra Ireland. It's the national organisation for people with EB. There's a Debra in nearly fifty countries: the UK, the US, Australia, across Asia. Our contingent grew out of those early days, with that little group of us sitting side by side with our parents.

Debra Ireland isn't just a charity. It's a lifeline. It keeps us connected to research, treatment, politics and each other. It gives us focus, but also fun. It gives us a calendar, things that we look forward to, events that we all attend yearly – the Kerry Challenge, the Butterfly Ball. With Debra Ireland we are part of something larger.

I can honestly say that Debra is where I found myself. And I don't mean just the public side of me – the speaker, the fundraiser, the person in the photo with the government minister. I mean the me that existed outside of hospital beds and dressings. The me that laughs my head off even on my worst day. The me that *hopes*.

It's funny to think it all started in a corridor with a little girl who didn't know she was being watched, sitting there on her mother's lap swinging her legs, trying not to pick at a bandage, probably wondering if she'd get to have something nice for a treat in the car on the way home.

* * *

Among the other children who went to Dr Watson's clinic were Bobby – the little boy from Limerick – Aaron, Fallon, Cora, Patty, Stephen and Adam. They were children I only saw once a month. I don't think we ever met outside the clinic, and we didn't send each other birthday cards or meet in the park. But still, once a month, we'd all be there – same place, same time – and it meant something. It was a special connection.

There was one little child I'll never forget, whose face and body were both badly affected with relentless EB. This child lived with their grandmother because they needed extra support. I didn't know all the words the adults used when they would talk about the situation with such sadness, but I *knew*.

One day we were queuing to be weighed – the child, suffering from desperate wounds, was in front of me. And I whispered to Mom, 'I'm lucky,' because I could see the difference, not just in our skin, but in our spirit.

Mom squeezed my hand. 'Poor thing's given up, pet.'

And she was right. That child passed away not long afterwards.

Maybe they didn't want to fight any more. Maybe they didn't have the strength. Honestly, I couldn't blame them. EB is hard enough without other burdens.

I held Mom's hand tighter that day, grateful for her and for my life in Abbeyleix. And for the fact that she hadn't given up, and I wasn't giving up, and for knowing neither of us ever would.

* * *

I used to cry in my sleep as a child. Mom would sit up with me, singing me a lullaby, stroking my head or holding my hand until I settled, still in terrible pain but too exhausted to stay awake any longer. Thank God for sleep.

Sometimes when I'd settle, Mom would crawl out of the room so her footsteps wouldn't wake me. Sometimes she would only get as far as the door before I would start crying again.

I remember lying so many times with my head on Mom's lap and her gently rubbing my forehead in soft circles. Sometimes she was singing, but sometimes she was quiet, not saying anything.

My mom has never failed to sit with me when I needed her to do that – not just because I was in pain but for everything else. Every now and then I wonder if this has been worse for her than for me. She has had to harden herself in ways I can't even imagine. Her job is to protect and comfort, and there have been many times she has been unable to do either. She had to watch people actively hurt her baby and she had to do it too. All the time. She is an amazing woman.

If you've ever seen me in person, you'll know I wear bandages on my arms, my legs, my torso. It's part of the routine for EB, but it wasn't always. I only started wearing bandages around the age of eight, as soon as my mother heard about them as a treatment.

Before that, the medical advice to EB patients was simple: avoid injury. That was all they could offer. Just, don't fall. Don't bump into things. Don't wear the wrong thing. Don't roll over in bed. Don't sit down too hard or for too long. It sounds impossible, doesn't it?

Even today, dermatologists give us some advice on skin care, but the bottom line is this: be careful of yourself. That *is* the medical guidance.

Mom and Dad did everything they could to keep me safe. But I could bump off a chair or catch my ankle on the leg of a table, just like anyone, and I'd be in agony because my skin tears like wet tissue under fingers. It wasn't just hard on me – it was brutal for everyone who loved me.

At around five or six I had a major fall on a little garden path in my aunty Martina's house in Sligo, where my mother was standing. I had been playing up above with my cousin Sally Anne, and Mom didn't realise I had come down behind her. She stepped back, knocking me off the path into the rockery. I was, of course, terribly wounded and my poor mother felt awful. That is EB: normal mistakes and normal actions have terrible consequences. It was an appalling reality for me and for my parents.

There was another time when I was being minded in my aunty Angela's and I got my fingers caught under the door. It's something that happens to most children at one point or another. Of course my fingers were totally skinned by it and poor Angela was devastated. My mother tried to explain that accidents happen and that this was the bargain we all struck when they took me home – I could not be protected from life. But Angela cried over it anyway.

As a sufferer of EB, I don't go a day without a wound of some kind. Not then, not now. The risk of infection is constant. Keeping wounds clean and dry isn't just a nice idea, it is literally survival. Many people with EB die from sepsis. Sepsis happens really fast and usually it isn't caught until it's too late to do anything. Most of the time, the infection spreads and creeps through the whole body silently, and it gets you that way. People think they have a stomach bug or the flu, but they're actually dying.

When I was little, my mom used Cicatrin powder to keep my wounds dry, which you can get in any pharmacy. Some people used cornstarch, others baby powder, but we swore by Cicatrin. It helped to keep my wounds dry most of the time, but not always.

One winter I was at my Nana Fogarty's house and I had on a little dress and tights, like most small girls wear around Christmas. Tights were usually fine for me. But as I was playing around, whatever way the tights were, they caused friction and wounds. As if that wasn't bad enough, when my mother went to take them off, they had adhered to my wounds. They were sealed on and stuck into the open sores.

My poor mother had no option but to peel the tights off, bit by bit. Each pull peeled skin too, and I was left with no skin below the knee. I don't remember the pain as much as I remember the look on my mother's face. It was a look I've seen again and again. It's a look I still see sometimes. A look of steel, like she has to switch her heart off in that moment. Because that is the truth – she does. For my whole life my mom has had to hurt me terribly, over and over again, just to care for me.

I also sometimes saw a look of helplessness and guilt, even though nothing of this is her fault.

When you're little you fight tooth and nail against every procedure, and paediatric nurses can end up having to hold you down in operating rooms. I remember having these awful plastic masks pushed onto my face and resisting as the mask filled with putrid-smelling anaesthetic gas and I experienced that horrible feeling of being overtaken by it. I still feel terror at just the thought of it. But in every memory the voice of my mother is above the clatter of my feet and the whispered instructions of the nurses, crying out to me so I would hear her, 'I'm here, Emma, you're alright pet, Mama is here.'

She could have run away, she could have waited outside. Yet, even though she could do nothing to make it all better, she stood right there. If she couldn't help, if she couldn't fix it, she would be there. For me.

I'm so grateful to my mom for putting me first in those moments. I'm so grateful for her stoicism and bravery in those operating rooms and surgeries, when she probably wanted to pick me up and run away.

Mothers are programmed to comfort their children, but mine so often had to go against that instinct to keep me alive. She never failed to be strong.

* * *

One of my favorite photographs of my mother and me was taken when I was in my thirties. My friend Jude had secretly nominated Mom for a Hidden Heroes award and I was nominated too, so we kept Mom's nomination – for the Unsung Hero Award – a secret until the last minute. Catherine and I gently encouraged her to wear this stunning lemon dress, just in case she had to go up on stage. I wore green.

I remember crying down the phone to my aunt Angela, both of us hoping with all our hearts that Mom would win. Because no matter how often I tell her, or how much she knows it, there's something powerful about public recognition. Awards like that show the world what it really means to be the parent of someone with EB: the constant sacrifices, the love, but also how much of a fight parents have to get the support they so badly need.

When we finally told her what was going on, on the morning of the awards, the first thing she said was, 'Do I have to make a speech?' But I could see how touched she was.

Mothers are so taken for granted – they give up everything for their children and no one stops to recognise it. But I see it. I see every bit of what my mother has done for me. She gave me life, and then she helped me really live. There's no award that's big enough to show how grateful I am that God sent me to Pat Fogarty.

4

All Too Well

Doctors sometimes remark that EB wounds are similar to third-degree burns. Burns are the worst injuries for skin. Burns are another time when skin can tear away under pressure. If you've ever had a bad one, you'll know the feeling.

The difference is that your burns heal, your skin scars and gets better, and your pain eventually goes away. For me it never does. Just *being* is painful. Just sitting down, moving to wake a dead leg, turning in my sleep is enough to break the skin. The parts of my body that press against chairs – my bum and my thighs – they're always wounded, always open and raw, like burns.

I live with never-healing, never-ending wounds.

When my skin tears, we try to gently place it back, hoping it might hold. But it rarely does. Every shift or movement in my seat will tear it further. Then it's back to square one. Another wound, another thing to manage.

When I was really small, we had nothing to cover the wounds. We would just wait and hope that things would get better. Mom dealt with each wound as it came, and hoped for new and better treatments, keeping in touch with other families and listening to advice from anyone who had gone before me.

The family we knew in Limerick, with their little boy Bobby, had gone to London and they were using a new system of care for their EB child. Bandages. 'It acts as a scaffold for his skin,' Bobby's mother told mine; my mom went straight to Crumlin Hospital and asked – begged – for access to this new system.

'That's only in the UK,' she was told, 'we don't have that here.' But Mom would not take no for an answer. She kept asking and, eventually, we were referred to Great Ormond Street Hospital in London.

We flew over as a family and stayed for a few days, meeting with their dermatologist and his team, who did a full review. I saw physiotherapists, dieticians and dermatologists. They took biopsies, which were just as brutal then as they are now. Then they wrapped all my wounds in bandages. My mom watched closely, learning each layer, each fold, which cream to apply, which gel went first, how to keep it snug but not tight.

'The gentle pressure of the wrap,' the doctor told us, 'gives the skin more stability. If refreshed every couple of days, the bandages will act as a barrier against the bumps and knocks of normal life, as well as infection.'

'Let's try it, Emma,' Mom said. She knew it was right, but I, barely eight and a half, needed real convincing.

I remember walking up and down the hospital stairs for the team. Going up was okay but coming down it felt as if the bandages were restricting my feet, and I was terrified of falling. I shuffled down one step at a time, gripping the railing.

'What do you think, Emma?' the doctor asked me.

'I don't like it,' I said.

That was how I felt. I didn't want to wear them. I told everyone. I told Mom. I told the nurses. I told the doctors. I just didn't see the point. It was uncomfortable and, anyway, I was used to the way things were. Like most kids, I didn't love change, even when change was for the better.

'Take them off!' I insisted, 'I don't like it.'

I could not get used to this.

***

We stayed in the hospital for three days. The results of the biopsies came back and we found out what kind of EB I had. Recessive dystrophic EB.

They introduced us to the Milton bath – an antiseptic soak to reduce infection. The water burned like nothing else. Wounds and water are a cruel combination, as anyone who has ever had a cut or scrape will know. But having clean skin is crucial. Mom would lift me into the bath, wash me and dry me as I cried, and then get to work applying each bandage, slowly and carefully.

Bandages back then weren't what they are now. They were rougher. I don't know how I ever let anyone put them on me, but they worked. The process was similar to what burn victims get: a layer of burn gel, then a cream, then thick cotton wool, all wrapped tight with layers of bandage.

After the few days of feeling that extra bit protected, that little bit safer, I finally saw that this *was* better. So I would sit still while Mom wrapped me up, as she had been shown, at home. From then on, she did most of my bandage changes as a child. She became an expert.

It was trial and error in the beginning. Sometimes they'd send the wrong size. Sometimes we'd mix up which bandage went on which body part. Then Mom would have to take it off and start again. It takes hours, but she never rushed or lost her patience. She never put it off until the next day. My mother always carried on, quietly and lovingly, doing what needed to be done.

The bandage routine changed our lives in good ways and bad

ways. Going from a kid with a basic bath routine to that kind of intensive care was a shock. It was hard. I remember sitting there, holding onto my mom's jumper as each bandage was wrapped.

I won't make light of the ordeal that a bandage change was and still is. Bandages hurt like hell going on and they kill coming off. I have to do partial changes daily and a full body change every second day. Without them I would – at this stage of EB – be bed-bound at best.

Yes, the routine takes a lot of time to do, but it is worth it. Bandages let me go out and about. Bandages let me *live*.

I will always wrap my skin, even though it's painful and so tiring. I do it because I'm protecting something valuable. Me. My body. My life.

The only day we don't do them is Christmas Day. That's the rule. I get Christmas Day off, where it's just the four of us with our prosecco and presents and total peace. I get one day a year without it. That's it. *One* day. Every other day, no matter what's happening, the bandages have to be done.

We take a selfie every Christmas. It's become a real Fogarty tradition, just us, no bandage change just one beautiful day off and total peace. I treasure those selfies.

At eight years old, about 40 per cent of my body was affected by EB. That's 40 per cent of me wounded all the time. That sounds massive, and it was, but compared to now, in my adult life, where it's 80 per cent, it feels like a time of innocence, and thank God for it. Back then, my face and neck were mostly okay. Anywhere without friction. It's friction that kills the skin. So I was wrapped just where I needed it.

Now, I'm wrapped nearly everywhere.

* * *

EB is a condition that gets worse progressively. I was born with the condition and for the first part of my life it wasn't a deteriorating illness. I had EB and it was manageable. It was never worse than it had been before. Until I was eight.

At eight, it seemed I started to move off the plateau I had been on since birth and my body started to struggle in new ways. My skin became more fragile. EB spread to my throat.

I'd never had a problem with food before. Then, suddenly, food was getting stuck. It started with a square of a fruit and nut bar, something I'd had a hundred times, but that day it got completely jammed in my throat. That soon became routine every time I ate. I'd cough and splutter, terrified, totally unable to swallow. My parents would give me water, terrified themselves. I mean, they couldn't even pat my back. They definitely couldn't shake me. So I stopped eating because I became too scared of choking.

My weight plummeted.

'Emma needs more weight on,' Dr Watson would say in our clinics, and my mother would explain that I was still refusing to eat. My weight was a constant topic of conversation in that clinic. I was always the skinny child. You can see it in photos – I look like a gust of wind might knock me sideways.

Eventually they sent me for a barium test.

I don't know if you've ever had to swallow barium, but it's like drinking liquid concrete. As a child, already afraid of food and barely able to swallow what I did like, it was unbearable. The nurses were as kind as they could be, encouraging me. But I still had to drink the stuff myself – they couldn't do it for me. I cried and begged the whole way through it.

The tests showed that my throat was scarring internally. The space food had to pass through was narrowing.

'Food will continue to get stuck,' the gastroenterologist said, 'it could get worse.'

So we started to limit what I ate. I'd have soup or mashed potatoes or yoghurt. Plenty of ice cream, which I was delighted about.

But even then, I would still choke. By the time I was eleven the doctors were insistent that something must be done.

'The risk is,' they said, 'that Emma's oesophagus might close completely if we don't do something now.'

Hearing that, everyone agreed to try to fix it and I had my first throat surgery to stretch the scar tissue and give me back some ease in swallowing. They slid a tube down my throat under general anaesthetic and tried to repair it, but it didn't work. In fact, it made things worse.

I couldn't speak properly after the surgery and I couldn't eat at all. I was kept in hospital for days, barely able to lift my head. The healing process was slow and painful. Things did improve slightly for a time, but then the scarring came back. So they tried again. This time the relief lasted barely a month.

The horrific operation became routine. Every three months I would be brought into surgery and I'd go through the entire process to stretch my throat again. That became my normal. It was like a reset button, but with worse side effects every time.

The resident EB nurse in Crumlin, Ursula, used to ask me after surgery, 'What are you looking forward to eating now, pet?' I'd usually say, 'My Christmas dinner.'

By the time I was fourteen they decided the time had come to do something new. My throat was getting worse, but I couldn't keep going as I was – scared to eat, losing weight, running on empty. EB is hard enough, but when you don't have all the vitamins and minerals and calories you need, it thrives.

People with EB have to be in the best health so they can fight off infections.

I needed a solution.

The dietician talked to us about a PEG tube – a permanent valve in my abdomen that would deliver food into the stomach directly. It wasn't a complete fix – even though it would sort out the problem of nutrition, I would continue to need the throat operations. It was also a serious operation, but we really had no option. We had to agree or leave my life on the line. It wasn't an easy decision, but we knew it had to be made.

After the operation the pain was unreal. It was horrendous. I couldn't sit up, I couldn't speak with it. I cried non-stop for days.

The team warned me to be mindful of the tube. 'You could knock it out,' they warned. So I became obsessed with checking it and we rushed to hospital more than once, thinking it had moved.

In time, I adjusted. I made friends with it, this little lifesaver. I even gave it a nickname – 'the button'. It became part of me. It kept me going. I was grateful for it.

I got all the nutrition a girl my age needed straight into my stomach. I didn't try new things, I barely ate, but I was healthy at least.

Getting the PEG tube marked a change. Now I was fully medicalised. And once you cross into that world with EB, you don't really come back.

Eight was the last year when my condition was fully manageable. It was the last year when I was simply 'fragile'.

After eight, I started to have to fight for life.

5

We Are Family

I don't know if there was a weekend when we didn't go down to Limerick, because my parents came from there. We would mostly stay with Nana Fogarty, but my mom still had family down there as well: her mother, brother Tom and sister Marguerite. My mother saw her other sisters regularly too; they would be up and we would be down to their homes now and again. But Limerick was home base, so we would all be in great form going down, my father especially, whistling and singing along to the radio.

Nana Fogarty lived in a big, warm farmhouse that was surrounded by fields with cows. When we arrived on Fridays we would drive around the side of the house and into the back yard, where cows stood with their heads over the wall, their big noses moving as they chewed away. As you got out of the car you would smell the dinner through the always open window.

Everyone went in the back door of that house – the front door was only for strangers. There were always cows and there was always a dog. Nana had poodles, but for some reason I don't remember those so well. I do remember one dog she had, Zent. A black and white pointer, he was bigger than me!

There was a big milking shed in the yard. When you were outside, the huge door would be a pitch-black hole. It scared me a bit, so I always played over the other side of the yard. I remember one time running into a billy goat out there who chased me – I barely made it inside safely.

Nana's husband passed away when my dad was only five. I think that was how they formed such a close bond, as she had to run the farm herself after that and he was the eldest. Later she took in a farm hand who lived with her, Jimmy. He was a soft-hearted man who Nana fed and minded because he had no family. He did most of the farm work then. I used to bully Jimmy to play snap with me, and he would always relent and play while keeping one eye on the news, which was great for me because it meant I won most of the rounds.

Like most Irish farms in those days, all the activity revolved around a big kitchen table where people would sit, eating or taking a cup of tea before they carried on with the hard work that farm life dictates. Nana's was the hub for my dad's side: his brother Tim-Joe, who was married to Aunty Catriona, and my dad's sister Phenie, short for Josephine. Tim-Joe and Catriona had four children: Edwina, Joe, Hazel and Katie. Edwina is the eldest grandchild on dad's side and I'm second. We were good pals when we were small, and we would play cards together on the floor of Nana's kitchen or walk around the yard gabbing about whatever. My cousins knew they could rough and tumble with each other but needed to be more careful of me. I loved seeing Tim-Joe's car when we would pull in at Nana's, because it meant that Edwina was already there and we could play.

Nana's kitchen was split with the sitting room on two levels – there were two or three steps from one to the other. There was no sofa in the sitting room, just armchairs that were set around a big heating range. They were those old-fashioned Irish armchairs with patterned fabric and wooden arms and legs, mismatched and lined up as if to say come in and sit down. There was a really old TV in the corner by the range that the chairs all faced. In the kitchen, when you went back up the few steps, there was the big table and my nana was always there, checking pots and ovens for whatever meal she was making – invariably meat and vegetables. There were always sandwiches as well, and pots and pots of tea.

In the evenings, if you were looking for me, you'd find me on Nana's lap, when she would finally sit down to watch the news and whatever came after. I used to play with her thumbs, one in each of my small hands, making them go around each other. She never stopped me from messing with her hands like that. They had soft, wrinkled skin and short nails – farming women's hands – and I loved them. I loved her voice when she would call out to the cows to take it easy, or to the dog to stay. Or when she would call me and my cousins to come in for dinner.

Nana was one of a few people my parents trusted to mind me, even when I was really small, and she had developed a knack for picking me up. When I was small, Nana would carry me around as she did things, which I loved. She never hurt me.

Every Christmas she would buy me a winter coat, a 'good one' to last to the next year. It was such a highlight to get that coat. I still keep up the tradition now – I always buy a new coat for Christmas, even though I'm obviously not growing out of the last one and have a wardrobe full of them. Can you ever have too many coats? Can you? Really?

Nana was only sixty-four when she passed away. I was eight and I woke up to the commotion of my poor father receiving the news. It was the early hours of the morning and his brother had called to tell him. We got straight into the car and drove all the way to Limerick in silence. My father's shoulders shook as we got closer to the house. When we pulled in, there were cars parked everywhere and the house was full of people. So it was true.

Nana was laid out in a coffin in her bedroom and people came in and out of the room as the Rosary ran in loops and the priest came. My parents stayed in there with Nana, while I went in and out with my cousins. I don't think I really got it, not until I went in and saw the undertaker closing the lid on the coffin.

I started crying out for them not to, begging them. 'No don't,' I said, 'please don't close it. Nana … Nana!' My voice echoed what everyone else was feeling inside.

My mother took my hand and brought me out. She sat me down beside my cousins, and Edwina tried to distract me.

A few weeks after Nana passed, I was asleep in my parents' room when my mother switched on the light – she needed to get something. As she pottered around, I lay there and I saw a halo forming around the soft light of the bulb. In it I saw my nana's face appear. She was smiling at me. I watched her as she faded away and then I went back to sleep.

The next morning, I told my parents.

'I saw Nana,' I said, as if it was the norm, 'she was in the light.'

My dad, still deeply grieving, asked me to tell him all about it. He asked me a few times. My story stayed the same each time. I was certain then and I still am. I did see it. I remember it so clearly, my nana's love reaching out to me one last time. I think it gave my dad comfort to hear it, and it definitely gave me comfort, both then and now. I think she was telling me she was okay. Maybe she was telling me I would be too.

The piano in our house once belonged to her. I played it

as a child. It's a lovely reminder – not just of Nana, but of my childhood full of light and music.

After Nana's passing, we stopped going to Limerick as much. We still visited on the odd weekend for a while, but the farmhouse had lost its heartbeat and gradually those visits got fewer and fewer. It was too hard on my dad. So I lost touch with Edwina and my cousins and saw them only on special occasions from then on. But we are still family – that never changed. I have little cousins once removed now too, as my first cousins have all settled down with their own families. There is Chloe, Adam, Odhran and Rhys, and Tomás and Katie's little boy, Tadhg.

6

Castle on the Hill

For me, the rites of childhood didn't come so easily. Sports days, fun runs, tug-of-war, I always stayed on the sidelines for things like that. Or home altogether. But look, I never even asked to go most times. I *knew*. Mom didn't have to give big explanations. She'd just say, 'No, not that one,' and I'd understand.

Primary school was, for the most part, sweet and wonderful, and I'm so glad. I never felt left out. And that's down to my parents. They never made a fuss or gave big pitying speeches. They gave comfort and good advice instead.

The way my mother was, I knew a 'no' was for a good reason. Because she had made that pact with her little baby all those years before. I knew if I could do it I *would* do it.

All children fall, all children get badly cut and skin their knees. But when I fell, when I hit my knees, it meant real damage and weeks of recovery. If Mom said 'no', it meant the risk just wasn't worth it.

There were moments – watching other kids playing or doing things – where I would think, *I'd be good at that.* I have always felt able-bodied inside in my soul. From the time I was small, when I would watch my classmates playing rounders, climb walls or do wheelbarrow races, I could almost feel myself right in the middle of it, strong and fast and tumbling around without fear. But that longing – if you'd call it that – would soon pass. I knew the rules.

I did get to do after-school activities, just not the sports variety. I did speech and drama, and every year I would try out for the Feis. One year, I read a prayer. You were meant to kneel during it, but I couldn't. So I sat on a little chair, said the prayer clear as a bell and with as much holiness as I could muster. I ended up coming second and my parents were delighted. You'd swear I'd won an Oscar. They kept the medal for years, proud as anything. I bet if I asked for it, they'd still be able to dig it out.

I got to do the school plays. Those things gave me a way to be part of some action at least; one of the few times I could join in and be like every other child there. I wasn't running races or doing cartwheels, but I could stand up, say my lines and feel like I belonged.

And I did belong. In primary school I was one of the gang. I remember my first crush (of many!), a boy in my class. I told someone my secret, I don't remember who. I must have been around ten. As tends to happen, she told someone who told someone and, before I knew it, on the night of the school play I walked in to a cheer of 'Tell him, tell him!' They made me sit up beside him on a table and I pretended I hadn't a clue what they were on about at all!

When I think back to those years, what I remember most is my parents' steadiness. The sense that even though the world outside was too dangerous for me, the world inside, in our house, was warm and predictable. I had my routines, my books, my quiet toys, my little wins. I had my dad with his chalk-covered jumpers and his funny ways. I had Mom with her soft warnings and her fierce love.

We always had dogs at home, we still do. But we had one dog I especially loved, the one who was around when I was little: Sam. He was a springer spaniel, you know, the kind that bounces off walls until you throw a ball. I loved him to bits and he seemed to understand that he needed to be gentler with me than he was with other people. He would bounce all over my dad, but with me he was softer and quieter, going down on his belly so I could rub him and following me around. I used to go out into our garden with him, and I would try to play tennis, holding the racket by the triangle part just under the frame with the handle resting against my waist. I'd hit the ball that way and Sam would go after it and bring it back to me.

* * *

When I was around seven, I was nominated for the Child of Achievement Award, through Crumlin Hospital and McDonald's. My teacher nominated me. I don't remember much about it, except the special dress I picked out with Mom (the beginnings of a lifelong obsession with *guna*s) and I remember sitting with another EB family, Val and Maria Fynes and their boy Aaron, who was a little bit older than me.

As we sat enjoying each other's company, Aaron leaned over to me and said, 'Will you marry me, Emma?'

I looked at him. 'No.'

This was very amusing for everyone there, but I didn't get the joke. I just remember thinking that it was absurd.

A couple of years later I went on the school tour. Of course, Mom was reluctant to let me go. I was still so little and wounds were so risky, but the teachers would keep an eye on me. I would stay the whole time with them, they promised. When she finally agreed, I swear I barely slept with the excitement. It was my first time going farther away than the bottom of the hill without Mom.

So you can imagine the stress for my poor mother when – in the days before mobile phones – the bus broke down on the way back and I didn't arrive home when I was supposed to. Mom was up the walls. She says it might have only been an hour late, but, for her, it felt like forever. The poor woman.

That was the beginning of my adventures away from Mom. A year later she let me go away overnight with Ursula, our specialist EB nurse in Crumlin Hospital. Ursula had heard about a two-night trip for children with EB that was happening in the UK, at Alton Towers.

'I'll take Emma,' she said to my mom.

We flew into Manchester to stay in the themed hotel. At breakfast, the characters came round – big-headed mascots – and I got my picture taken with every single one.

In the park, we went through the Haunted House and it was thrilling. Convinced of my own bravery then, I decided I'd go on a ride. I don't know what possessed me, but the one I picked was the Pirate Ship. You know the one – the giant boat yoke that swings you into the sky and back again like it's actually trying to throw you out.

I held on to Ursula and screamed the whole time, begging her to get them to stop it and let me off. It wasn't hurting me, it was just far scarier on board than it had looked from the sidelines. Jackie, another nurse who was there, kept saying, 'You're alright, Emma, it'll stop now,' over and over.

Eventually it did. I bolted the second it slowed.

Having not learned anything, I then went on another ride – that big robot-arm thing that spins you in circles. I got wounded on that one. It wasn't worth it, but I was glad I'd tried. I never went on anything as crazy as that again.

It was when I was around nine that Mom brought me to an equestrian centre not far from us that held classes for children with disabilities. It was run by a lady named Anne O'Halloran. She had gathered some little ponies there that were used to children, ones that walked softly and took their time.

I remember, as we pulled in, looking at Mom as if she had lost her mind. But she had been down to check it out without me and she had seen how safe they made it for all the children who rode there.

The pony I rode most often was a brown, furry Shetland pony with a thick mane. I don't remember his name – I wish I did. I wore the smallest helmet they had, but it was still too big. I had two girls beside me, holding the reins on either side, and one girl walking backwards in front of the pony, speaking to it and to me calmly. It felt like I was part of a little team. Mom was so nervous, I could see her trembling every time I looked over.

Some kids would go off riding on their own, trotting or even doing little jumps. Not me. I never rode alone. It was those three girls, the pony and me.

The first time I went they encouraged the pony forward into a trot and the helmet on my head bobbed around far too much. I was convinced it was going to take my forehead off and so I begged them to stop. Another week a pony started acting up and bucked, throwing its rider to the ground. I remember the fear in me watching, because her foot caught in the stirrup when she fell and for a moment she was dangling. I kept thinking that was going to happen to me too.

'Do you want to try a trot, Emma?' they'd ask me every

week, and after that incident I'd look at them like they were attempting murder. 'No way,' I'd say.

I really didn't want to go faster. I loved being up there and it was enough. I loved the sway as the pony walked along. I loved the soft thuds his hooves made in the arena and the earthy smell of the straw.

* * *

My childhood was so sweet. At home, I had a huge wooden doll's house filled with wooden furniture. My best friend from school, Orla, used to come over and we'd play with it for hours. We'd rearrange everything again and again, making up stories about the dolls and their lives – all drama and minute details.

Orla and I sometimes had minor rows, the way all little girls do – when one has the Barbie the other wants, or when the other won't hand over the tiny hairbrush. You know the way. Orla would sulk or I would sulk, but it would never last long. We always made up. Those little tiffs never lasted longer than a moment or two.

Our whole class was like that. We'd known each other so long, we were almost like siblings. Some of my primary-school friends – Kathy, Bernadette, Shane, Rory, Patrick and Liam – are still people I see all the time. When Kathy lived in Dublin, she would always drop in if I was in hospital with a book for me. And Bernadette did a fundraiser for EB in her lovely shop – I was so proud of her for that.

I was such a happy child. I think about that a lot, because people expect the opposite. They think I must have been lonely, or sheltered, or desperate for what I couldn't do. The truth is that when you're loved, when you're safe, you don't miss the things you've never had. Not in any devastating way at least. And when something is given to you – like a bike, or a pony, or a class of children who treat you like anyone else – it feels like more than enough.

There was never a moment where I suddenly realised I was different. I never had any big *Oh God* realisation. It was just I added it all up over time. I wasn't like Mom or Dad. Orla could fall and get up again, no worse off. Most kids' mothers didn't have to drive at a crawl to avoid potholes because one knock might land their child in hospital. But it didn't hurt to understand this. I was happy.

What my childhood taught me was this: there's a work-around for nearly everything. I wanted to ride a bike, and I found a way. I loved animals, and someone helped me ride horses. I couldn't run, but I could still move through the world in ways that made me feel free.

That's how I try to see the world now. Not through a lens of lacking, but of possibility.

It's why I get excited when I see ramps being built, or new tech being designed, or even just a shop that's thoughtful about how it lays out its space. These things matter. They tell people like me that we're seen. That we're worth the effort.

I didn't get to keep cycling. I didn't go galloping through fields. But I got to *try*. And sometimes, trying is everything.

Sometimes, it's enough to just ride in a circle, gently, with three girls walking with you, and a brown pony who seems to know just what you need.

Sometimes it's enough to cycle only downhill, to feel the wind in your face, even if it's just for a minute.

7

The Best Day

Catherine was born when I was ten. I'd been hounding Mom and Dad for *years* to get me a brother or a sister, like they could just pop down to the shop and pick one up. I probably thought they could, in fairness. Babies came from hospitals, didn't they? Well go get one!

I wanted someone permanent to play dolls and cards with – but I hadn't exactly considered the ten-year gap.

Mom says I used to ask her over and over, 'Can I have a sister? Can I *please* have a sister?' She'd say, 'Maybe someday,' or 'We'll think about it.'

Of course they had been told not to have any more children. With the recessive gene, the chance of having a baby with EB is one in four. Doctors thought that was too big a risk.

But Mom had always dreamed of having a big family. And when she met my dad that is what they'd planned. The house they bought as newlyweds had more than enough bedrooms.

I don't know if my badgering had anything to do with it, but my parents eventually decided to have another baby. Although the risk was there, they decided to take it. Mom told me years later that she worried the whole time, but they had decided that if another baby came along with EB they could handle it. They would get help and hire a nurse.

Thankfully Catherine was not a one in four. She doesn't have EB.

* * *

I followed my pregnant mother around like a second shadow, watching her bump grow. She had this jumper she used to wear all the time – it was grey with a brown bear on the front. The bear had red mittens or maybe a gift in its hands, I can't fully remember now. But I remember Mom in it. I remember her hands holding mine to her bump so I could feel the baby kick.

Limerick were playing in the All-Ireland hurling final when Mom started pacing with labour pains and told my dad they needed to go. The match was nearly over and Dad, sitting nose to screen in his Limerick jersey, was *almost* about to ask her to hang on.

When they opened the door to bring her bag out to the car, my aunt Marguerite was coming up the driveway, there to catch the end of the game with my dad. My mom remembers thinking this was bad timing, but Irish manners are Irish manners.

'I don't think I can see you ...' she said, wondering if she should put the kettle on, 'I'm in labour, I might have to go.'

Marguerite didn't so much as set a toe in the door. 'Just go, Pat!' she told my mother.

So we all piled into the car, me already in my pyjamas, Mom in pain, my dad stressed out (probably as much for the match). The drive to Dublin was a bit frantic. Catherine came quick – as second babies often do – and I remember at one point Dad said, 'I might have to pull over and call an ambulance.'

But we made it. *Just.* I was dropped off at Aunty Angela's and put straight to bed across from my cousin Aoife. I was confused. Even though I knew Mom was having the baby, I didn't understand why I couldn't be there with my parents for it. I had thought I'd go with them to help. Sure, I could hold it in the car on the way home, couldn't I? It was my idea after all!

This was the biggest thing that had ever happened to our family and I was left behind. It was very confusing and I was raging.

'Go asleep, Emma,' my aunt whispered, seeing my eyes glistening in the dark when she put her head around the door. I turned my face to the wall and closed my eyes, and the next thing I knew my aunt was whispering, 'Emma, pet, you have a little sister.' My cousin Shane was there too, beaming.

I can still feel it when I think of that moment. That warm shock in my chest like magic.

'I'm happy,' I said.

'Go back asleep,' Angela told me. *Yeah right.* I lay in the dark feeling that magic flood through me. I had a little sister.

As soon as the sun came up, I got up. I somehow knew my dad would be in Shane's room. I don't know how, but I ran straight there and found him, curled up and turned into the wall. I tapped his arm.

'Daddy,' I said. He turned over, sleepy but smiling.

'Can we go see the baby, Daddy?' I was straight on this.

'We will, pet, after breakfast,' he said. Instantly, I had his covers back and was pulling his legs off the bed. If that was the case, we would have breakfast right now.

Downstairs I took one bite of toast, then stood up. Dad made me eat a few more bites before giving in, then off we went to see the baby in Holles Street.

I remember a long corridor that went all the way around the

hospital and I ran the length of it, way ahead, with Dad calling after me to be careful. I was desperate to see this new sister of mine. I peeked through every door until I saw Mom sitting up in bed, fussing into one of those little plastic cribs beside her. That's where the baby was. I ran straight over.

I wasn't strong enough to hold her properly, but I wanted to try. Mom sat me on the bed, laid the baby on my lap, and we held her together. I looked down and thought, *She's mine*. I'd asked for her. I'd waited for her. And now she was here. I don't think I've ever felt prouder in my life.

* * *

When we brought Catherine home, she slept in my room for a while and, listen, I took my role very seriously. If she cried, I was the first to respond – unless it meant getting out of bed fast, which I wasn't always able for.

One night she started crying, so I gave her my brand-new teddy – a Teddy Ruxpin – the one that sang songs when you squeezed him. He was my favourite toy at the time; I think Santa had brought him.

Catherine stopped crying and held the teddy tight, and that was that. He was hers now. He ended up with a new name – Sleeping Teddy. I had Sleeping Dolly. A little duo for a little duo.

Unfortunately, Sam got to Sleeping Teddy and had him torn open in seconds, with the musical part ripped right out. That bear was just fluff and threads when Mom found him.

I was heartbroken, but Catherine lost her reason.

Mom didn't panic. She got a tea towel, the sewing kit and went into full doctor mode.

'We'll fix him up,' she said to a sobbing Catherine. She talked to the teddy like he was a real patient. 'Don't worry, Sleeping Teddy, we'll get you sorted.'

She was performing a little play to calm us down. And it worked. We watched the operation very seriously.

I saw how Mom loved everything we loved. Nothing was too small for her to care about – not even a battered teddy who'd lost his voice.

Sleeping Teddy never sang again. But he stayed and so did the feeling that Mom gave us that day. That said to us the world might be tough, but our family is soft. That said things are not always perfect, but we have each other. The message that told us firmly that love could be sewn into the very seams of things – my baby clothes, this poor Sleeping Teddy.

* * *

When Catherine was able to stand, I devised a way to lift her out of bed in the morning, so I could be the one to get her up. I'd get her to wrap her little arms around my neck and I'd wrap mine around her back, and I would spin her gently sideways and onto the floor. To put her back, I'd spin gently again and sort of launch her onto the bed.

Mom was baffled when she saw it the first time.

'How did she get out of bed?' she said, staring at us.

'I lifted her,' I said. I was so proud. It made me feel strong and sisterly.

There was a time Catherine gave us all a scare – she ran into an open lift that shut behind her in a hotel where we were on holiday. Mom ran upstairs. Dad bolted for the lobby. I was left alone, something that rarely happened, but I couldn't enjoy it. I stood there, scared out of my mind. The lobby opened straight out onto a main road, if she came out down there … it didn't bear thinking about.

Mom found her eventually, after a woman tipped her off that there was a small child playing away happily one flight up. But for those ten minutes, we were frantic. I will never forget the relief of seeing her in my mom's arms.

Someone asked me recently if Catherine always knew I was fragile. The straight answer to that is, eh … no. She did not. She was a baby. So she pinched, pulled hair, smacked, shrieked and generally did what babies do. Mom and Dad would try to tell her, 'Be gentle with Emma,' but what baby could grasp that idea?

I remember one time I was lying on the couch, my hair in a ponytail, and she came up and twisted a chunk of my hair so tight it came clean out of my scalp. I screamed. My parents ran in and there Catherine was, delighted with her fistful of hair. It took my parents ages to get her to let it go.

It hurt like hell, but I was secretly delighted in a weird way. Not about the hair, obviously – but because this baby treated me like any baby treats their older sister.

As she got older, she started getting the idea. My wounds and bandages – those weren't normal sister stuff. She finally understood that I needed extra care and she stopped smacking me or pulling my hair.

Catherine brought a bit of wild into our house. Before her, things had been calm and careful. Our life was predictable. Then came the swings and the slides in the garden. One for her, and one specially made for me, with a back and sides.

Not only that, but she brought our extended family such a sense of newness and fun. Her older cousins adored her as much as I did, and the younger ones were delighted with their new playmate.

We live in a bungalow, and whenever we would go to my aunty Angela's, Catherine would bring every single teddy she owned (a lot) and line them all up on the stairs. It was her favourite thing to do.

Once, our dog had puppies, and as soon as we saw our cousins, Catherine came straight out with it.

'We have puppies,' she said with a proud face.

'Oh yeah?' my cousin Aoife replied. 'Well … we have stairs.'

Catherine fell apart at that. I think she would have swapped those pups for stairs on the spot.

When she was five or six, I was doing my Junior Cert. I had to make a clay butterfly for my final project in art and I was really struggling with it.

'Take a break, Emma,' Mom said, and so I did. But when I came back to it, it was in pieces.

Catherine had tried to help me and, in her enthusiasm, she had broken part of it. When she realised it was damaged, she tried even harder to fix it and completely ruined it.

She was nowhere to be found at first, but when I did find her, I will never forget how upset she was at what she had done. It made me really upset to see her so upset. I couldn't have cared less about the butterfly when I saw my sister so sad.

Now that we're adults we hang out. We're friends. Proper ones.

We've had our rows, like any sisters. But there's a bond there that was stitched in early.

I got what I asked for. A little sister. A best friend. Someone to pass the teddy to.

I am so grateful that Catherine got to grow up without pain, without dressings or hospital stays. There has never once been any part of me that wished I had a comrade in EB. Because I wouldn't wish this on anyone, least of all her. Even if she did pull my hair!

As a baby, and as a woman, Catherine has never seen me as 'her sister with EB'. She has only ever seen Emma.

8

The Outside

I never had any idea that there was another pain in life. I didn't know about the hard side of emotion. I'm so grateful to my parents for that. I'm so grateful to my wider family for that too. As a small child my only hardship was EB.

Primary school was filled with little restrictions, but my whole world to that point had been gentle and so sweet. And I am so glad I had that experience, where I was sheltered from the other stuff – conflict and mind games. I had been kept from the psychological pain that comes with being recognised as different.

Then a new girl joined our class: Lorna. And she was ready to let me know all about it.

She arrived when we were heading into sixth class, but the rest of us were still the same little kids we had always been. Lorna was from the city, with the cool confidence that comes with it, and she knew all the latest bands and songs and TV shows that we didn't or were only catching up on.

'Dolls are for babies,' Lorna said when I asked if she wanted to play.

'Do you not watch MTV?' she said as if we were all from the moon.

Even to my innocent eyes, Lorna was cool in the worst kind

of way. Even the way she carried her schoolbag, barely slung on one shoulder, was with edge. She would give you a look too, a once over that I had never seen before but that instantly made you feel small and unsure of yourself.

To my dismay, on meeting Lorna, Orla's eyes lit up and suddenly she was over there instead of over here. Suddenly she was talking about MTV and things I'd never heard of. Suddenly she was going out to play in the yard instead of staying in to play with me like always. She didn't even put her hand up to volunteer to stay any more.

There I was on most familiar ground, feeling like a total stranger. I had no idea what to do.

Mom did.

'Maybe the trick,' she said, soothing my upset with softness, 'is to make friends all together.' She rang Lorna's mom and invited Lorna over to our house after school the next day. Lorna did come, but she was hours late and, unfortunately, when she arrived, my mother said to her, 'Oh, we had a few tears thinking you weren't coming.'

I wished the ground would open up and swallow me. The look on Lorna's face when she heard that was one of utter disgust. I knew the story immediately: Lorna had not wanted to come over, she had resisted. She was being forced. I showed her my Barbie house, and I showed her our dog, but she just sat on the sofa and stared into space until her mother came to get her and she could go home.

* * *

Mom had heard of a great dressing for kids with EB and we were trying it out. It was a cling film-style burn dressing and it didn't absorb. I wore it for a while, but as the day went on and my wounds reacted with the cling film and the heat of my skin, it gave off a strong smell. I don't think I realised, but Lorna made sure I knew about it soon enough.

'Emma really smells,' she said to Orla when they were standing right near me. Orla's face flushed and she looked at her feet.

I went home and insisted to my mother that I wouldn't wear those dressings again. The new comfort wasn't worth *that*.

That was the final straw for me. I wasn't in a trio. I wasn't even really in a duo any more, not in school anyway. Orla still came over to play in my house. But in school she didn't know me. If I called her, she would look my way with a faraway expression, as if confused to hear her name. If I spoke, she would act like there was nobody there.

I don't want to paint myself as a saint. I'm sure I had ways that rubbed people up wrong. I don't expect everyone to like me and it was clear I didn't make the cut with Lorna. But Orla and I had had such a bond. That's what made it sting so much. It wasn't just losing a friend – it was losing *her*.

We'd had plans, Orla and I. We were going to go to the same secondary school, sit beside each other, do homework together. But once Lorna came along, even talking about the future changed. If I did, even at my house, Orla would look away and go quiet. I could feel the shift in her.

Then Lorna made it clear. 'She isn't your friend any more,' she said one day. Just like that. I'd gone looking for Orla, hoping for a game or even just a chat. Instead, I got that. So I stopped asking. I was too afraid.

Everyone's had that moment, haven't they? The friend who drops you for someone else. We all remember it. I'm *almost* glad I had that experience, because it made me understand and connect with other people. On loneliness. On heartbreak. On cruelty. These things that are so common they're practically a rite of passage.

I just wish it hadn't been Orla who taught me about it.

Anyway, Orla's mother started making excuses to mine about why I couldn't come over, or why she couldn't. I overheard them once, talking about secondary school – Orla and Lorna – and they had plans I wasn't part of. That was the nail in the coffin.

I asked Mom if I could go to a different secondary school altogether. Anywhere but there. Sadly, the only other option was too big, it wouldn't have been safe for me. My other friends were going there, but I *had* to go to the smaller school as planned.

The last day of sixth class was emotional for everyone. We all stayed back after the bell, crying like our hearts were breaking. And maybe they were. We all knew it was the end of something good.

I sat there, crying quietly, knowing that this wasn't just the end of primary school. It was the end of that version of my life. I went from being a child who *loved* school, one who skipped in the gates and waved at every face, to someone who counted the minutes until the bell.

* * *

Walking in on my first day in secondary school was like walking the green mile. As these children pulled away from their own childhood, they pulled away from compassion and lost the gentle understanding that little children seem to have built into their bones.

Orla and Lorna teamed up and I walked around alone. My class didn't have one little room where we could be all day, we didn't have one teacher we knew and loved. There was no place for me to stay behind at lunch because the timetables shuffled us from one room to another.

I'm not going to sugar-coat it – I really suffered with bullies from that time on. Unfortunately for me, Orla and Lorna were not the worst of it.

There were, of course, moments of light. There were always, year in, year out, one or two people who made space for me when no one else would. My guardian angels of secondary school, that's how I think of them now.

Jackie Cuddy was one. She was in her last year of school, sixth year, when I was in first year. I remember her spotting me shuffling along alone at lunch time and I think she suspected I was being isolated. She would sometimes come down to find me at lunch and bring me down to the hall to play badminton. This was a gift to me, that game, because I could play it. I could hit it, run (a bit), laugh.

Jackie never treated those games like charity. She played with me and then walked me back to class as if that was exactly what she wanted to be doing with her time off. I've never forgotten her. And I never will.

The rest of the time, I was on my own. I had no friends, not even in the familiar faces that walked by me linking their arms throughout the day. But wow, I tried, in those early days. Believe me, I really did. I'd approach the girls from my year at lunch and try to chat. I would think as hard as I could about what to say that would slide me into their conversations. I wanted what everyone else wanted – people to sit beside, people to laugh with. But my attempts never landed. They looked through me like I was invisible. And, unfortunately, callousness is contagious in teenagers.

People always remark offhand that children are cruel, but I've never agreed with that. Children are *honest* – they're blunt, but they don't start off wanting to hurt you. Children will ask me, 'What's wrong with you?' or 'What happened to you?' as easily as they will ask why the sky is blue. And they mean it – they want an answer. It's not malice. It's curiosity.

Children never frame their questions to deliberately hurt me. They aren't acting ignorant just to twist the knife. It's teenagers who do that. It's teenagers who are cruel on purpose. They *learn* how to wound. They *know* where to aim.

And in those years, they aimed at me.

Orla's friendship with me was well behind her and this new world of teenage apathy was louder, shinier. She took on the slinky looks and bubblegum snaps that the new gang did – Lorna front and centre with her loud voice and sharp tongue. Orla rarely so much as looked at me.

And I – totally unskilled in social manipulation – would try to speak to them. I would speak and nobody would respond. Just ... nothing. Not a glance. Not even a dirty look. That's what really got to me. It was like I was invisible, and I started to believe it. I was worthless and maybe they were right to ignore me.

I know that's not just how kids are. Because I was a kid at the same time. And when I had my little shred of social power – which I did during those battles in primary school to stay in with me at lunch – I never used it to push someone else down. *Never.*

There was a path around the school yard, a kind of gravelled loop about the size of half a football field. At lunch, if the weather was good, girls would walk it in a loop. The path was uneven and my balance was never great, but I would try to walk with them. EB slowed me down, I'd always been weaker. On top of that I had to be careful not to fall. So, after a few minutes, I'd start to lag, and when I fell behind, the girls never stopped. Nobody waited. They'd even lap me with linked arms and chatter as if they couldn't see me. It was so cruel.

It wasn't only that – there were the nasty comments as well. One day, it would be Lorna's loud voice behind me: 'Don't you hate when people sit where they're not wanted?'

Another day, it would be one of her gang turning to me mid-sentence and snapping, 'Don't be so nosey, Emma.'

If I sat beside them, they'd whisper. If I sat somewhere else, they'd call out across the room, the bus or the footpath, 'Emma, why did you move?'

'Why aren't you sitting with us?'

'What's wrong with you, Emma?'

Always that mocking tone. Always that twist of maliciousness disguised as friendliness.

I'd say, 'I'm fine,' trying to keep the wobble out of my voice. And they'd shrug and turn back to their whispering, satisfied.

The goal wasn't to get a reaction. The goal was to make sure I felt it.

I did.

* * *

Lorna was on the same bus home as me. Every day. And every day she chipped away at me on that bus. It wasn't enough that she pinned me to the board every day in school; she would go at me again on my way home.

Sometimes it was subtle – holding back a laugh, or a look passing between her and another girl. Sometimes it was louder. She would say something like, 'Isn't it terrible when people don't know they're not wanted,' and the others would giggle, and I'd know it was about me.

Once she was sitting on the lap of an older girl, Assumpta. They were being loud and showing off, and Assumpta leaned in and whispered something in Lorna's ear. She shook her head immediately and I saw a blush creeping up her neck.

'I can't say that. I'll get in trouble,' Lorna said.

That sentence stayed with me for years. *I'll get in trouble.*

What was it? What was so awful she couldn't repeat it? I'm sure it was something childish. 'Tell her to get off the bus.' Something like that. But it didn't matter what it was. The only reason she didn't say it was to avoid trouble in school.

There were always things like that – little flickers of self-awareness in the people who bullied me. They weren't monsters. They knew what they were doing was wrong. You could see it in their eyes sometimes, the way they'd look at each other sideways, unsure whether to laugh or not, like they were standing on the edge of something but couldn't resist jumping.

They'd push each other forward – 'You say it', 'No, you say it' – and then stare at me like it was all a big joke they were about to let me in on.

There was never a joke, of course, and whatever they were pretending to whisper about wasn't real. I knew that. Deep down I knew all of this had nothing to do with me and everything to do with them – their boredom, their fear of being different, their desperate need to belong.

Still, they made me feel the weight of it every single day.

They made me feel, for the first time, the social weight of my illness. And that gave them such … glee.

I was dealing with so much already. The bandages, the constant pain, the energy it took to get through a day – I didn't have the mental space to fight back. Even if I had, I actually didn't know how. Maybe I should blame my family for that. We never operated like this, not even for one second. I've never understood where that sort of thing comes from, because I have none of it. What type of life do you have to have to want to isolate and bully someone like me?

I don't know. Because even on my worst day, when I am wailing out loud and wishing the pain would stop for one minute so I could sleep, I am never cruel.

I still had hope back then, that maybe tomorrow would be different. Maybe tomorrow someone would say hi, or sit beside me. Some days I would get desperate and try to make friends again, but every time I got burned. I got smaller and smaller. I became quieter and quieter.

But that still didn't stop them.

I was in the first-year locker room alone when one of Lorna's gang came in – one of the worst. She found me, squatted down in front of me like I was a child, looked me in the eye and said, 'Look Emma, I don't want to tell you this, but … everyone thinks …'

And the dagger went in, in, in, deep into my exhausted heart.

I won't write what she said. I won't immortalise it.

I sat there, bandaged, in pain and exhausted, and I nodded and said, 'Okay.' That was all I could manage. I didn't know how to tell her to go away. I didn't know how to say, 'Leave me alone.'

Oh, I feel so protective now over the child I was – I wish I could go back and stand behind her, hand on her shoulder, and speak for her. I wish I could fight back for her.

But I can only do that now, here, with words.

9

Invisible Strings

On my mom's side, there's Uncle Tom, married to Joss, with their kids, Roger, Gareth, Sonia and Derek, who sadly passed away. They're a good bit older than me. And I have my aunts, Marie, Marguerite, Angela and Martina. They all watch out for Mom. Maybe that's because she is the youngest.

Aunt Marie married Billy, who passed not long ago. He was a real gent – sharp as a tack, never afraid to speak his mind and always in my corner. Marie and Billy had Shay, Mark, June and Margo. I saw them a lot growing up. We all have that cousin bond still, where you might not talk every day, but when you do, the years just drop away.

Marguerite has always been a quiet presence in my life, showing up just when she is needed.

Aunt Martina married Charlie, and they had three children – Yvonne, the eldest, then Cathal and Sally Anne. Sally Anne was just a year behind me. We were thick as thieves when we were kids. Every summer, we'd pack off to their house near the sea in Sligo for a long weekend. We'd walk down to the beach with our buckets and play.

Then there's Angela, married to Sean. Her children are Nicola (married to Dan), Shane (married to Bethan), and my cousin-slash-big-sister Aoife. Aoife's married to Gavin – one of life's good ones. He never treats me like I'm fragile, just as I am. I was really unwell for their wedding, and it was one of those times when I got so frustrated with this disease. I had bought an amazing royal-blue dress – I'd had it made specially – and I was so looking forward to it all. I remember sitting at the dinner and I wasn't able to eat or drink. Then, all of a sudden, I knew I was going to be ill and I got sick into a napkin. I caught a waiter's eye as I sat back up, and he looked so uncomfortable. I turned to my sister and said, 'Catherine I have to go.' We went outside and the minute we did, I knew something was wrong. I was so cold. Catherine got me water and I went up to my room thinking I would come back down, but I never did. I was sick all night. I was so disappointed to miss the party and not be able to celebrate with Aoife and Gavin. Now they've got the twins, Evie and Cian, who are eight.

Like Aoife, Nicola has been like another big sister to me. She always comes to visit me regularly, as does Aunty Angela, when I'm in hospital. They are so supportive to me and the whole family, and I am beyond grateful for them. Nicola even drove down to the house during Covid to deliver a desk to Catherine, as she didn't have one big enough for her to work from home on. I was at Nicola's wedding last year and it was a really special day for everyone.

Shane and Bethan have a son, Sean. They gave me the honour of being his godmother on my twenty-first and I have watched him grow into an amazing man. They have a beautiful girl too, Ellie.

We are a very close network, our family. I honestly could not have made it without every single one of them.

And of course there was Nana Bowen.

* * *

My mom's mother was small and delicate, with tiny hands that were as white as her hair, which was pure white in contrast to my other Nana with her dark-grey hair. Nana Fogarty was someone you climbed up on. Nana Bowen was someone you peeped through the crack in the door at.

Nana Bowen's skin was soft and smooth, and the way she moved gave her this magical air. She used to walk so quietly you'd never hear her coming. She floated around in a world of her own, almost completely deaf. When she spoke, however, that bubble was burst as her deafness caused her to shout. She always had Fox's mints and boiled sweets in a tin with her, and I'd sidle up and shout loudly right into her ear, 'NANA, CAN I HAVE A SWEET?' And she would bellow back, 'YES, PET,' and then fuss around getting the tin out and open with her dainty little hands to let me choose. I always went for the red one.

Mom and her sisters had an arrangement where Nana Bowen would live a month at each of their homes, changing over somewhere midway between their houses. So, we would drive to Mullingar or wherever and collect Nana, who would then come to stay in the spare room. I loved the little journeys to Mullingar the most because, once there, we would all have a coffee together with Nana before she would come back with one of us. It was a really wonderful routine as it meant we all got to have the experience of living with our nana.

Nana Bowen had so many grandchildren she couldn't buy each of us an Easter egg, so she used to buy a load of Creme Eggs instead. It was the same every Easter, and I would be hopping in anticipation of getting that egg above all of the other full-size chocolate ones.

'HAPPY EASTER, EMMA,' Nana would roar and press it into my hand.

The value system of children is never straightforward because the Creme Eggs were the eggs we all looked forward to the most.

One night the fire alarm in our house went off, scaring us all to pieces. It was when Mom was pregnant with Catherine, but she bolted out of bed and turned all the lights on thinking something must be on fire. I ran up the hall after her, not knowing what on earth was happening. Well, we found Nana Bowen sitting right there in the hall smoking a cigarette under the fire alarm in her nightdress. Mom had to take the cigarette away and stub it out, then put Nana back to bed, and then me.

Another time, when Catherine was around two, we were on our own in the house, with Nana Bowen supposedly asleep in her bed. We were watching telly sitting on the couch. Well, Nana appeared suddenly at the door of the living room, and she was so pale with her white hair and white nightdress that Catherine and I both screamed the house down. Nana wasn't fazed by that at all – sure she couldn't hear us.

Nana Bowen was in hospital when she passed away. I was in bed and Mom came in very late one night and told me she wouldn't be there in the morning as she had to go to see Nana Bowen.

I remember asking over and over, 'Is Nana okay?'

But all Mom would say was, 'I don't know.'

So I asked, 'Will she get better?'

Mom answered, 'I don't know' to that question too.

'Can I come?' I said.

'No, Emma,' Mom said, 'you stay here and I'll see you in the morning.'

But Mom didn't come back in the morning because Nana passed away.

Her funeral was at my aunt Marguerite's house in Limerick. I remember going in to say goodbye to her before they closed the coffin. I was in the room with all of my cousins the same age as me – Sally Anne, June and Aoife – as we lined up to say goodbye to our nana. After saying goodbye, we ran out of the sitting room one by one. I was the last. I was following Aoife down to one of the bedrooms when one of Mom's friends stopped me and held on to me. I was already bawling crying. But I remember, even in that moment, thinking: *I don't want this person hugging me. I want to be with Aoife. I just want to be with my cousin.*

That's all I have ever wanted – to be with my family.

* * *

One of the most dramatic moments of my teen years was when my mother, Catherine and I were driving back from a Dublin hospital appointment and we crashed.

We were coming through Monasterevin at the time. Mom always drove so carefully and slowly with me in the car, especially around corners. Anyway, we came slowly around a bend near the Hazel Hotel when another car came out of nowhere – at top speed – and slammed into ours, sending us right across the road into a stone wall. What we didn't know in that moment, thank God, was that the wall we had disintegrated with our car was the edge of a bridge. If the impact had been harder, if Mom hadn't been crawling along, we would have definitely gone over into the stream.

When our car came to a stop, I froze. Mom started screaming. She couldn't see Catherine. For one horrible second we both thought something awful had happened. Then we heard a little groan and realised that, in the tailspin and impact, Catherine had been flung sideways. The force of the crash had thrown her from her car seat, sending her across and downward. The poor little thing was now under the front seat, wedged there.

'Get out of the car, Emma!' Mom said, and I scrambled out like the car was about to explode. Mom got out and pulled Catherine out. The man who had hit us was making his way across the road, and his face was red and horrible.

'Get away from us,' I shouted, and I hit him with a balled fist; 'Just get away.' He didn't argue. He backed away.

Cars stopped and people came; someone called the gardaí and they arrived and rang Dad from the scene. They gave Mom the phone and my poor dad heard an explosion of myself, Catherine and Mom crying into the phone.

'Daddy,' I remember sobbing, 'please come help us, Daddy.' He did. As fast as he could.

The ambulance came for the walking wounded, which at the time *I* saw as Catherine and Mom. Catherine had a little cut on her nose and Mom's neck was hurting her. All I had was a cut on my forehead from hitting the dashboard. Yet everyone was treating me as if I was the worst off.

'I'm fine,' I said. I wanted them to see to the baby and to my mother.

Once we arrived at the hospital and the nurse cut off my jumper, I realised why there had been that sense of urgency around me. My white shirt was soaked and dark with my blood. The seatbelt had torn the skin completely away from my abdomen, my elbows were shredded, the skin on my shoulder was gone. All that time I had thought I was fine, but I wasn't. I was wrecked. The adrenaline was powerful, it had kept me from feeling the unbelievable pain.

'She's hit her head,' one of the doctors said. 'We need to monitor her for concussion and take care of the wounds.'

They told Mom I needed to stay in hospital, but Mom looked at them like they were mental. 'That wound's from EB,' she said, 'not the crash. I can care for Emma better than anyone here, at home.'

They looked at her – at me – then understood.

'Well,' the nurse said, 'she needs to stay the one night in case of concussion.'

Mom agreed to that, and she took Catherine home while Daddy sat up all through the night with me. I had nothing with me, so I slept in my tights.

On the way back, we passed by the hotel and pulled in to see the car. It had been towed into the car park of the Hazel Hotel, the same one we'd passed moments before we were hit. It was crushed and completely caved in at the front. When I saw it, my stomach dropped. That car looked like no one should have walked out of it. We were so lucky. There's no other word for it.

After the crash, the nightmares started and they were awful. The crash played over and over in my dreams and there was always this scream – one scream.

One night I was asleep, dreaming about it again – the car, the scream, the panic – and in the middle of that dream I woke up, heart racing, skin clammy. Because I'd heard the scream, but this time it wasn't in my head.

Mom had fallen outside on the step. Her scream matched the one from my dream exactly. For a moment I didn't know if I was still dreaming or if I'd woken into something worse. Mom was fine, but I shook for the whole day.

Thankfully the nightmares faded, but the memory of the

crash has stayed with me. The sight of the crushed car. The sound of Mom's scream.

There was a court case after a few years over the crash. Not a full trial – just a session in the courthouse where a judge read through settlements and approved them. I remember being in the hallway and hearing, 'In the matter of so-and-so versus Emma Fogarty ...' Then the clerk said something like, 'not to be given before her eighteenth ...' That was it. They moved on to something else.

I don't remember the figure, and the money went into a bank account I couldn't touch until I was eighteen. All I remember was thinking at the time, *I want to be eighteen right now.*

During the day in court, I left the room at one point to go to the bathroom, and there was a man standing in the corridor. He didn't say anything, but he stared at me and watched me the whole way from the courtroom to the bathroom. I don't know if it was him – the driver – but something in me said it might have been.

10

Mean

By the end of second year in secondary school, I'd given up on believing I could ever have friends. I kept my head down. I'd sit in the canteen on my own at lunch, watching groups of girls laughing and chatting.

But I never stopped wanting it.

They saw me as a way to bond with each other. They would concoct tricks and humiliations for me all the time. Like the time one of them came up to me as I was sitting on the steps of the school hall at break. The gang huddled a little way away, watching.

She held something out to me in her hand. I ignored her, knowing full well from experience what this was.

So she waved it closer. It was an unfurled condom from a packet.

'Do you know what this is, Emma?' she said.

I said nothing, I just stared into space. That always worked when they pulled this sort of thing on me. Eventually she would go away.

'Do you know what to do with this, Emma?' she said, and she looked back over her shoulder for encouragement before she brought the condom closer to me.

I came up with a great answer in my head. In my head I

said, 'I do, do you need me to explain to you how to use it?' But I didn't say it out loud. I was too afraid of her, of them. I said nothing, I just stared into space, so she laughed loudly and walked off.

* * *

My form of EB is not just blisters and wounds. It's arthritis. It's osteoporosis. Injuries, with EB, just happen. You don't have to fall, you don't have to be hit hard, sometimes one small misstep can cause your bones to break. I have been plagued with trouble in my bones all my life, especially in my weak foot, the left one.

I was born with that foot torn to shreds. The umbilical cord had wrapped around it in the womb and actually skinned it. So that particular foot always plagued me. It's always where the skin went first, always where the bones would let me down. I'd spent years going in and out of Dr Watson's office because of that foot in particular – my literal Achilles heel – and it was always in pain. A constant gnawing pain I couldn't ever seem to dose away. I'd lived with it.

So we'd be doing dressings and Mom would ask, 'Which one's sore, the little or the big?' And I'd say, 'The little.' It was just how we talked about it.

I would actually title this book 'My Left Foot' except it has been done already!

The first time I broke my foot was in fifth year, and it was the first time I experienced life from a wheelchair. When I went back to school after time off over it, the class head came straight up to me at the start of class and plopped an envelope in front of me. Inside was a card that said something like, 'Hope you feel better soon' on the front. I opened it and saw all the signatures

– the same girls who blanked me, bullied me, walked past me every single day like I was nothing. The same girl who had waved a condom in my face. The same ones who laughed and whispered.

I saw names I didn't want to see – Lorna, Orla – side by side.

I sat there and let silent tears drip onto the table. That card affected me in a way I hadn't expected. Either they were hypocrites or I had it all wrong.

And I *knew* I didn't.

That hypocrisy took on a pattern.

In secondary school I had two sets of books – one for school, one for home – but I still had to carry them between classrooms. The school bag I used to carry them around in rubbed my shoulders raw and left me in tears some days. There were no lockers and no allowances made for me in secondary school.

Anyway, one time I was going up the stairs and I think because I was concentrating on the bag so much I didn't watch myself and my little foot missed a step. I fell forward and hit my head.

My bully from the bus, Assumpta, was passing by as I fell. She stopped and started cooing at me, then lifted me onto her lap and sat on the floor there in the middle of the corridor holding me. She meant to look compassionate, maybe she genuinely wanted to help, but to me it felt humiliating. I couldn't struggle or shrug her off, I'd have hurt myself, so I just kept asking her to let go. I didn't want to be babied. This girl had her face posed like a saint the whole time, while completely ignoring my requests to be put down.

I was either not there at all, or I was an excuse for girls to virtue signal or get out of what they were doing.

Mom used to drive me to school in the mornings, but I took the bus home. I never told her what was happening on that bus. I never told her I was being excluded. I don't know why.

Maybe I didn't have the words. Maybe I thought she couldn't fix it anyway so why should the two of us suffer. Maybe I just didn't want to see my sadness reflected in her face.

In the house, I had Catherine. My little sister didn't care about school cliques or bandages or whether I sat alone at lunch. She cared about getting her big sister to play shops. At home I was seen, I was Emma, I was a sister, a daughter, a cousin.

At school I was nothing.

Maybe butterfly skin made those young people uncomfortable. Maybe my bandages worried them so much they wanted to ignore them. Maybe they just couldn't cope with what I had to cope with. And so they shut me out.

But here's the part I cling to. The part that makes me love my younger self so much. *I didn't let them.*

I kept talking to them, even when no one responded. I kept walking that path, even when I knew they'd pass me and I'd be left behind. I kept trying. They saw that as annoying and irritating, but I know what that was.

I was holding on to my soul. I was holding on to my softness. I was holding on to my kindness. I was holding on to the Fogartys and the Bowens.

I wasn't falling for what these girls fell for: this idea that you have to be cool, that you have to be hard and callous to be part of a group.

That's something I'm really proud of now.

And you know what? All these years later, some of the girls who were the meanest to me follow me online. They've seen the things I've done, the causes I've spoken for. And sometimes they send a little message. 'You're amazing, Emma.' 'I remember you from school – you were so brave.'

And I smile. Because they *do* remember. And so do I.

I remember feeling hated and ostracised, I remember being in pain. I remember wishing someone would sit with me or talk to me. I remember catching snippets of conversations I would have given anything to be part of but never was.

I could name and shame, but the truth is I don't know most of their names because they faded into the background as soon as I left school. Life moved on and I got too busy living it. These days I rarely think about those girls. But the pain still sits somewhere in me, quietly. Of course it does. That little girl trying to make her way is still in there after all. But I don't carry hate – I don't have room for that – I simply carry the memory and I won't forget it.

Things did get a little better later, in fifth year, when Ashling came into our year. She wasn't afraid to speak to me and laugh with me. It was so new that for the first while I was suspicious of what she said and did. But then she pulled together a small group – herself, Thelma, Trisha and me – and for the first time in years, I belonged to something. We weren't close, but they made the last years of school bearable.

11

A Whole New World

My parents had been to Florida on their honeymoon. They totally fell in love with the sunshine, the palm trees, the theme parks and that all-American smile you get from people, even when they're just handing you a coffee over a counter. They always wanted to go back, so once Catherine was old enough – around five – we did.

Florida was magic. I was around fifteen when we went for the first time of many. The second time we went, the following year, I was starting to use a wheelchair. Since breaking my foot, I used it sometimes when I got tired.

But the first time we went to Disneyland, I walked the whole park. Slowly, with lots of stops, but I did it. I loved walking through the place more than I cared about going on the rides. I loved the big pastel buildings, the pretend castles, the characters – it made you feel like you were in a storybook.

Even at five, Catherine was flying ahead with Dad to get in the queues for the huge rides – that's them always. But when we caught up it turned out that Catherine was too small to go.

'You're not tall enough,' Mom told her gently, but Catherine was having none of it. She had a bit of a tantrum, that's how desperate she was to do it all. Catherine's energy and resistance, I loved it. That's just her.

Me and Mom? We like a slow stroll. We are the ones stopping at every little sign to read it, popping into every little shop that comes along for a look, just because they're there.

I never go on roller coasters, but in Florida I saw one called the River Rapids. You might know it – a fast-moving river with huge blow-up rafts that sail along at speed. My dad loved anything that had speed and water as a combination, and that was his favourite. He would go again and again. What was so, so funny was that when he would get soaked, he would be absolutely raging about it. But he would dry off, forget the misery and queue up again.

I don't know what possessed me, but as Dad and Catherine went to queue for the River Rapids one day, I decided to go too. I was so scared I actually cried and, of course, I got soaked, which was never good for my bandages. But the sun dried them fast, thank God.

After that, Dad looked around for a gentle ride, so I could go on it too.

'This one,' he said, in front of a stand that had dinosaurs on the sign.

'It's a simulator,' he told us. 'It feels like a roller coaster but doesn't leave the ground.'

Well, I was battered on that thing. Poor Daddy felt so guilty; he'd been convinced it would be gentle, but it wasn't.

I did find a ride I loved, the Tea Cups. Spinning around was so fun. Unfortunately, Daddy didn't think so – after the third go he was almost sick with the dizziness.

'I'll stick to the roller coaster, Emma,' he said.

We had a ball in Florida. We went into all the mad cafés, such as Planet Hollywood and the Hard Rock Cafe. Those places are wild. Guitars hanging off the walls beside fake tigers,

Elvis Presley memorabilia next to T-Rex skulls. It makes perfect sense and no sense all at once.

We went to SeaWorld too. I remember lining up in the sun outside and a woman approached me with a little girl in a buggy, waving.

'Excuse me,' she said, 'do you have EB?'

'Yes I do,' I said, and I looked in the buggy and knew exactly why she was asking. Her little girl had it too.

'Her name is Hayley,' she told me. As we stood in the line together this mother asked me question after question. We gave her as much information as we could. I could see in her face this relief, almost, to meet someone older with EB, and in that small meeting perhaps she took away hope that her daughter could live with this and go travelling and be free.

I felt really blessed to have had the chance, a one in a million chance, to talk to that mother and meet Hayley.

* * *

We only ever took holidays in August because Dad worked correcting exams in June and July. So we always hit Florida at its hottest. It was sweltering. One year Catherine got heat stroke and collapsed in the hotel. It's no joke. Mom and I would duck into every shop we passed just for the air conditioning.

I think that's where I got my love of shopping, hopping into shops with Mom whenever it was too hot or too wet. We would spend time in there together, looking at absolutely everything, calling each other if we found something special.

I remember buying my Eeyore teddy one year. The little donkey with the stitched-on tail. I still have him, propped up on the head of my bed.

I always connected with Eeyore. He and I are similar. He always tries to be social when he feels awful.

Thankfully, the weather in Florida would cool down after it rained, and it rained *every day* in the afternoon. Catherine, being herself, would run out of wherever we were to dance and skip in the heavy downpour. She loved it. It really was a highlight of her day. While we would be sheltering in doorways and running into shops, Catherine would stop and spin and get soaked. I can still see her now in my mind's eye, her face turned up to the sky and her arms out dancing. She was so cute.

That sort of mentality that you see in Catherine, it comes from my parents and it comes from me. We really believe in making the best of things in the Fogarty house. It's important to us. Maybe taking me home from the hospital set this unwritten family motto in motion. We really do live in the moment as much as we can.

And in Florida we could do that in a way you didn't get to at home. Holidays are wonderful, aren't they?

One year we went to a water park that had a lazy river-style swimming pool running the whole way round it, and, with Fogarty spirit, I became obsessed with the idea that I would have a go on it the next time we went. Mom looked, had a think and bought me a wet suit that we rolled up over my limbs and my bandages. I was really excited. The lazy river was amazing, we all hung on to each other and floated along sat into our rubber rings, no drama. But by the time we got to the end I had become wedged into mine and couldn't get out. You can't really pull people up when they have EB, it's too dangerous. I was totally stuck and nobody could really figure out how to get me out.

Eventually, my dad very gently held my arms while a kind man (who was floating by and stopped to help) pushed down on the ring. Finally, I popped out, and Daddy carried me up the steps because I was in my bare feet. I was fine. Well, until myself and Mom realised that a wet suit does not keep you dry! What we had needed was a dry suit. My bandages were soaked. I'm still not sure if that was worth it.

I remember another time waiting for a lift when a group of Chinese tourists came around the corner to wait too. One of them was fixing her hat and accidentally boxed my poor mother in the face. Poor Mom was mortified as she held onto her face and tried to be polite as the woman bowed and apologised until she was blue in the face. The rest of us were trying so hard not to laugh, and as soon as we were out of the lift we roared. It is a story we still tell. We were in such good form on holidays, not even a thump in the head could get us out of it.

We went to Florida for five years in a row. We'd leave and already be planning the next trip. The place had that effect on us. It was that good.

Once we had seen everything there was to see, we started to go to Los Angeles.

12

Perfect

There are moments in life that take something from you. You carry on after them, sure, but a piece of you stays there, frozen in time, hurt and bewildered. I'll tell you about my worst ever time in school, and then I'll move on and hopefully leave that moment behind me here, on these pages, for good.

Our class was planning its debs. All the chat was about dresses and dates – who was going with who. The debs is an Irish rite of passage. It appears to be all fun, sparkles and excitement. But underneath all the organising, there's a sort of quiet judgement going on in that invisible teenage ranking system.

I knew I wasn't high on the list. But I was excited to go with the few girls who were nice to me.

Caroline was one of the most popular girls in our class and she looked like she knew it as she walked around with her little gang. Her hair was perfectly in style, her uniform hung off her like a designer dress. She had the latest of things, yet her attitude still stank. She was the kind of girl who could and would say something horrible but never get called out for it.

One day, Caroline was chatting with Thelma about the debs and the table plan and who was sitting where. I was over the other side of the room writing in my copybook when there was a lull in the classroom chatter – one of those famously brief moments when a room quiets suddenly, just as someone raises their voice to be heard.

And I heard Caroline.

'Thelma, come on, you won't want to be stuck next to Emma.'

I felt like the air was knocked out of me, like I'd been punched in the chest.

She didn't know I'd heard. Neither did Thelma. But I watched it all. I watched Thelma freeze, give Caroline this really hard stare, then walk off. That was something, at least.

Then everything snapped back to normal as if nothing had happened. When I saw Thelma later, she acted as though everything was fine.

But it wasn't. It was as if that line held all the weight of everything I had ever been through.

We finished up for the day and, as I was leaving school, I saw Catriona, a girl I knew from primary school, walking near me. She was in my year, but she did her own thing most of the time. I don't know what possessed me – maybe she represented a safer time – I asked her if I could sit beside her on the bus.

She said yes. Then she looked at me and asked, 'What's wrong?'

And I couldn't answer. I turned my head away, but the tears came anyway. I walked off quickly, embarrassed, ashamed of myself for crying in public.

But she followed me. She wouldn't let it go.

Of course, if you poke something fragile, it breaks. I did. The whole story came pouring out.

I told her what I'd heard. The words Caroline had said. I

told her I knew what people said about me, that I wasn't pretty or perfect.

'It's not fair,' I said.

She was shocked, but not in that way where people say, 'That's awful', and then change the subject.

No, Catriona *felt* it. And the following Monday morning on the bus to school, she went straight up to Caroline and told her what I had heard and what she thought about it. When I found out, I really wished she hadn't.

Immediately, a cyclone of bad energy started whipping around me. Word spread. Emma was talking about Caroline. The cyclone twisted. *Emma was telling people Caroline was bad. That meant Emma was really the bad one.*

By the time Mom dropped me in – those few minutes late to avoid the crowds – I was public enemy number one with the popular girls.

Eyes stared at me. I heard my name whispered over and over. The drama built and so did the case against me. I couldn't stop it, couldn't catch my breath. I couldn't get control of the narrative, couldn't explain myself.

'Take no notice,' one of the sporty girls, Sonia, said. 'You'll be fine if you take no notice.'

But how could I take no notice? I felt every single scowl, every single whisper.

One day I just fell apart. I broke, in the middle of class, with tears I just couldn't hold back. I ran out of the room.

As I passed, I heard one of them – one of the ones who'd stood by and watched it all – say, 'My God, what is *wrong* with her?'

As if they didn't know.

I sobbed pretty much for the rest of that day and for days

after. I couldn't stop crying.

'They get away with this because they're popular,' Ashling said and held my hand gently.

But I couldn't stop crying.

'I don't want to go to the debs,' I said, 'I want my money back.'

'I'm going to say something,' Thelma said, and at lunchtime she called Caroline out of the room. Caroline went so slowly and stared at me as she did. Thelma eventually pulled her out by the sleeve.

Everyone went so quiet, ears pricked.

'Show a shred of decency,' Thelma could be heard saying.

I peeped out and I could see Caroline standing there with her arms folded, eyes half-closed in boredom. Her jumper was halfway down her arm from where Thelma had pulled it.

'Honestly, Thelma,' she said, pulling it back up, 'I am so over it now.'

People always look for explanations for bullies. You hear it all the time: 'Maybe she was insecure.' 'Maybe she was going through something herself.' 'Maybe it wasn't personal.' 'You don't know what was going on at home.'

Well, I don't want to hear it. I don't *care*.

Because I was suffering. Every single day. I was walking in there wrapped in bandages. Walking in fighting pain. I was fighting to walk, to move, to breathe, to *live*. And all I wanted was what every other girl in that classroom had. Someone to sit beside.

Lorna and her gang had taken that from me. Caroline did as well.

And the others? The ones who stood by and said nothing? They're to blame too. For weeks after that nobody but the others in my little foursome spoke to me at all and that kind of silence – the *maybe someone else will step in* silence – is just as cruel. It creates a space where bullies can thrive. Because nobody stops them. Everyone thinks someone else will, but no one did.

Secondary school was a time I felt truly erased. Not because of my condition – though that was part of it – but because of what it did to other people and what it gave them: power.

And it wasn't just the pupils who took advantage of that.

* * *

I could never wear our school skirt. The fabric was too rough and it tore my skin just by hitting off it. It also showed too much of my legs and the bandages on them. So, in a compromise, I wore the soft cotton school tracksuit trousers instead of the skirt. On top I wore the shirt and uniform jumper. It was an arrangement my parents had made with the school. I had brought in a note and given it to the headmistress.

But it still caused me a lot of trouble.

You see, every single time this one teacher saw me, she'd stop.

'Emma Fogarty, where is your uniform?'

I'd explain, 'I can't wear it, Miss. I have EB.'

She'd nod. Then, in a horrific game of Groundhog Day, the next day or week she would stop me and say, 'Emma Fogarty, where is your uniform?'

'I can't wear it, Miss. Remember? I have EB.'

I brought in more notes from my parents. I explained again and again. Showed her my arms, my bandages, my skin. But nothing changed. If she saw me, she asked me. And I would have to stand there again and explain myself.

Eventually, I got a letter from Dr Watson, which I brought straight to the staffroom and handed to that teacher myself. She read it. Nodded. I thought maybe – finally – that was the end of it.

But that *same day*, in the corridor, she called out again: 'Emma Fogarty, where is your uniform?'

I had another teacher, who taught us maths. She would constantly accuse me of getting my dad to do my work. She told me that was the reason I wasn't being allowed to do honours maths.

'You're not doing the work yourself, Emma,' she said.

'Test me!' I said. 'I *can* do honours.'

So she did, and I got 100 per cent, so she tested me again, and again I scored 100. I think she tested me four times until she finally allowed me a spot in honours maths.

'The only reason you have good marks,' she said as she gave up, 'is because your father is a maths teacher.'

Okayyyy.

It was brutal.

Years later that same teacher came up to say hello. I wanted to say, 'Go away, you were horrible to me,' but I just smiled and nodded until she was done praising me with how well I've done.

No thanks to you, I thought.

There were never any exemptions for me. There was never grace.

If I didn't do my homework – punished.

If I was absent – 'Not good enough, Emma.'

If I needed a break – 'You'll have one when everyone has one, Emma.'

That still boggles my mind. That a child wrapped in bandages, walking carefully on broken skin, dealing with exhaustion, infection and pain, would be expected to function like everyone else.

But that's school for you. It's a harsh little society all of its own. A hierarchy that thrives on exalting perfection and punishing those who lag behind.

I did have one teacher I loved: Mrs Lynch. She was really kind to me, and if I was choking, all I had to do was put my hand up and she would nod at the door to tell me I could head out. Sometimes, if I didn't know the answer to something, I would put up my hand anyway and leave the class. The way I saw it was that I was suffering enough to get any small benefit I could from it. But she totally sussed me out, and she mentioned it to my mom at a parents meeting. I stopped doing it from then on, I was mortified!

***

School is a system. And it's often a brutal one. And it is overseen by another brute. The Department of Education.

Coming up to the Leaving Certificate, my parents applied on my behalf for the special dispensation for students with difficulties. They really felt like I needed a little extra time in the exams, and I did. I had studied as hard as I could in between bandage changes and hospital appointments and throat surgeries. But at the end of the day, I am in constant pain and so sometimes I can't think very well. It gets so bad, the pain fills all the space in my mind. I stall and pause and can't form words or thoughts or anything.

Nothing about my pain is different from anyone else's. Just because I've suffered it my whole life doesn't give me super strength to deal with it. So coming up to the Leaving, my parents wanted to apply for a time leniency to help me cope with that and to give me the best chance I could have to recall the information I had learned.

Their application was refused, the comeback being that EB was not sufficient to warrant an extension of twenty minutes. Yes, you read it right: two zero. Twenty minutes.

My mom and dad were rightly outraged and pushed on with an appeal. They had to go to Athlone to fight it out with the department. Finally, the twenty minutes were granted.

Mom was always thinking ahead and, coming up to the exam, she asked the headmistress if I could be seated at the back of the hall. It was coming up to the time when I would normally have a throat operation, and so I was choking on my saliva a lot. But I had to delay the operation until after the exams. We all felt that I needed to be near the door, so I could get out quickly if I started to cough. That thought was not just for me but also for the other girls. We didn't want to disturb them either.

So Mom went straight to the top with the request.

'Of course,' said the headmistress.

When I arrived for my first exam, I searched the back for my student number. The desks all had stickers on them with the student numbers of those assigned to them. I asked for help to find mine and it was located smack in the very centre of the room. The table with my name and number stuck to it was packed in the middle of rows and rows. There was no quiet escape from that.

With the added stress of course, I started choking before the paper was even handed out. I didn't know what to do. I didn't know if I was allowed to just leave or whether I'd be penalised. I sat there, frozen.

And then – a miracle.

The supervisor walked straight down the hall, lifted my desk – the whole thing – and carried it to the back of the room. He set me up there and gave me the space I needed. It took him one minute to do that. He also told the hall monitor to ignore me if I went back and forth to the toilet.

Kindness doesn't take much time.

The day I walked out of school after my last exam, I was smiling. The others were crying, hugging, clutching their bags to their chests like the world was ending.

Maybe, for them, it was.

Maybe they sensed it – that this was the last time they'd be top of the ladder. Maybe they knew what I was also beginning to suspect – that life outside would be bigger, scarier and less impressed by these girls who ran the classroom.

I wasn't crying. I left that place like a bullet from a gun. Gone like a shot.

13

Hero

I did go to the debs in the end.

There were a few reasons for that. I wanted to attend the event I'd waited so long for. The three girls I liked in my class were going. I'd picked out a silky burgundy ballgown in town with my mom and sister, and I couldn't wait to wear it.

I *was* part of the debs fairytale already. I just needed to ask a boy. And I knew who my first choice was.

We've all had *that* teenage crush. A boy, *that* boy, the one you see every day on the bus or across the yard. The one you never actually speak to, but who occupies so much space in your imagination it's like he lives there. That was one thing I can say I didn't miss out on as a teenage girl.

There were small ones along the way, but the first real crush I ever had was Paddy Moran. He occupied most of my daydreams back then.

Paddy went to the school down the road from us, a year ahead of me. He was one of those classic, good-looking Irish lads, brown hair and dark eyes, clean-cut, polite to adults. A rugby player type, though I don't think he played. He had a quiet confidence about him that made it feel like he belonged to a higher order of boy than the eejits that acted like monkeys on the bus on the way home.

Every day after school, Paddy would get on the same bus as me. And every day I'd get intense butterflies when I saw him get on. Even if the day had been dreadful – whispering girls, mocking glances, loneliness – a glimpse of my crush would always pull me up and out of it.

There were always students coming and going from our house because Dad gave grinds in the evening. Some local kid would arrive with the prospect of maths exams hanging over them like a noose and go straight into the dining room, where Dad would be waiting for them with a cup of tea and his notebook ready to sort it all out. I liked that about our house, the coming and going, the sound of my dad's voice explaining. I liked knowing my dad was someone people trusted to help them. And look, I was a teenager – I also liked the fact that there were often boys at the door.

One night I was at home when the doorbell went, and I went to the door as normal and opened it. There he was – Paddy – standing on our doorstep. I just gawped. Nothing came out of my mouth when I opened it. He winked and walked by me, there for grinds with my dad.

Paddy never did anything grand. He wasn't loud. But every day that boy would hold my bag for me when I was getting off the bus and pass it out once I got down.

And some days he'd wink when I said thanks.

Those were the days I lived for.

Paddy had a girlfriend, of course. But that didn't matter to me. Even after he left school, I still talked about him non-stop to my friends. I imagined scenarios where he was single and I was confident enough to ask him to come to the debs and, in the dream, he always said yes without hesitation.

Then one day on the bus, my new travel pal Catriona leaned

across and whispered the words that changed my life: 'Paddy Moran's girlfriend cheated on him.'

She took a dramatic breath. I could feel the moment stretch, like the pause before a firework. Then bang. 'He broke it off with her.'

I thought I might explode. The impossible now felt possible.

'I'll *have* to ask him,' I said. But I didn't mean it. I didn't have the courage. Still, we talked about it all the way to my house and then Catriona stood on the step and we went over it one more time.

'I'll ask him for you,' Catriona said.

'No!' I grabbed her arm like it was a lifeline. 'Please don't. I swear, I'll die if you do.'

She promised. Looked me dead in the eye and *promised.*

She rang me later.

'I looked up his number,' she said. 'I think I should just ring his house.'

'No,' I pleaded, 'don't!'

'He won't even be home,' Catriona said. 'I'll just ring.'

'Please don't!' I said.

A half hour later I was pacing up and down the hallway of my house, bricking it, knowing Catriona was busy calling Paddy.

I think I held my breath through the whole wait and when the phone finally rang again, I could hear my heart in my ears.

'He said yeah,' she said. 'He wanted to know why you didn't ask him yourself.'

'I was too embarrassed!' I squealed.

I couldn't believe it. He'd said yes. *Paddy Moran* had said yes. So what did I do next? I avoided him like the plague.

I was *terrified*. Maybe he'd forget. Maybe he hadn't meant it. Maybe he'd change his mind.

If I avoided him, I'd never find out which it was.

***

The morning of the debs, I woke up in agony. Of *course* I did. This is my life we're talking about. Nothing ever came easy. Not even a day I had dreamed about for years, not even with the dress and the boy and the hope that maybe, for once, things for me would go okay.

It was my foot. That foot. My weak spot that never failed to give me trouble.

I couldn't walk on it. Just putting weight down made it feel like it would snap.

Mom went straight into panic mode. Half of her was trying to get me to lie down, to rest, to cancel the whole thing. The other half – the part that knew her daughter – was already hunting for solutions. She called the doctor. He gave me strong painkillers and told me to stay off my foot for the day.

In fairness, they could've told me to stick pins in it for all I cared – *I was going*. Paddy Moran was taking me, he hadn't forgotten. There was absolutely no way I was missing it.

But I did what I was told and did as little walking or standing as I could until the last minute. I got my hair done.

'Did you hurt your head, Emma?' my hairdresser, Anita, asked me as she combed my hair.

'No,' I said.

'You've a small cut,' she said. I knew what that was. I'd been trying styles the day before and the clip had been too tight.

'Will you get my mom?' I asked and she ran outside.

A moment later she came back in. 'Your mom is crying in

the car,' she said, 'I'm going to give her a minute ... she said you've had the hardest day.'

'No,' I assured her, because I wanted to go so much, 'I'm grand.'

But I did feel for my mother.

Eventually, I was ready.

When Paddy pulled up outside the house, it really felt to me like I was in a film. He stepped out of his car wearing a suit and holding a corsage that perfectly matched the pattern on my dress. I don't know if he picked it on purpose or just got lucky, but either way, it felt like fate.

'I've been in London,' he said.

'So, are you home for a visit?' Mom asked him.

'No,' he said. 'I just came home for the debs, I'm off again tomorrow.'

My heart did somersaults.

We took photos in the sitting room and, for one, Paddy leaned across and kissed me on the cheek like it was the most natural thing in the world. I played it cool, but inside? Oh my God, I melted.

Catherine squealed when she saw the kiss and whispered something to Mom. Mom laughed and then said something quietly to Paddy.

'Would you like a kiss too, Catherine?' he said, and she ran over and lifted her cheek just like I had. That was so cute.

We got into Paddy's car, which he was going to drive to the school to meet the bus that was taking us all to the debs. He'd leave it in the village overnight. I was fiddling with the seatbelt when Paddy leaned across and clipped it in for me. I swear to God, I don't think I breathed the whole journey.

My parents followed behind in their car – to wave off the

bus with the other parents – and then we were on our way.

I remember feeling so proud to be with such a gentleman as Paddy was. He was just incredible. He chatted to everyone. He shook hands and said hello.

And every single time someone asked who he was there with, he answered proudly, 'I'm here with Emma.'

He didn't say it as an afterthought or a favour. He said it like it was obvious and the most natural thing in the world.

At one point he went to the loo, and Catriona came up to me, all low-voiced and serious. 'I can't find John,' she said. 'What if he goes off with someone else?' John was her escort for the night.

I realised that Paddy was taking ages and I started to worry about him too. But then we checked, and there the two of them were, standing in a little group, having a smoke. Like it was nothing.

Because it *was* nothing.

Bullying does that to you. It warps your sense of what's real. You can't trust it when people are kind. You start looking for the moment they'll change their mind about you. You can't trust someone to be consistent. That's what happens when your best friend acts like you're a total stranger practically overnight. That's what happens when your whole teenage life has been built on whispers behind your back.

You learn *not* to expect goodness.

So when it shows up, you think it must be a trick.

Later, the music started up – Enrique Iglesias, 'Hero', the song of the moment. Every girl there knew the words. Every girl there had imagined dancing to it with a dream boy under dim lights.

Would you dance, if I asked you to dance ...

I remember that moment like it's still happening. Even writing it now, my heart is speeding up.

Paddy put his napkin down. He stood up and fixed his bow tie. Then he turned to me and said, 'Emma, would you dance if I asked you to dance?'

I – of course – said, 'No way.'

But he just grinned. Held out his hand.

'Go on,' he said.

'No.'

'Ah, go *wan*.'

He kept going. 'Go on, Emma. You have to. It's your debs.'

Eventually, laughing, I admitted defeat and gave in. I stood up, my foot still aching but my heart absolutely thundering.

As we walked towards the floor, Paddy leaned in and asked, 'Can I hold you for it?'

'Alright,' I said.

'Grand,' he said, and he took my hand and placed the other one gently around my waist.

And we danced with the whole room watching.

For those few minutes, I forgot it all. My pain. The bullying. The girls who turned their backs to me as I'd walked into that hall. I forgot the whispers. I forgot fear.

Everything fell away.

It was just me and Paddy, my dream boy on the bus.

We got the bus with everyone home that night, both of us quiet and content with the sun coming up. At one point he took off his jacket and laid it over my legs to keep me warm. As we neared Abbeyleix, I went to give it back and he shook his head and said, 'Keep it.'

He pushed the jacket back down onto my leg and patted it.

Yes – Paddy Moran put his hand *on my leg*.

That kept me in conversations with my friends for months. Maybe *years*.

When the bus dropped us off at my house, Paddy walked me up the drive and, as we stood there, the goodbye paused. I think the bus behind us nearly toppled over with the sudden weight of every kid on board running to look out the window.

Paddy leaned in – just slightly – for a goodnight kiss.

And …

Mom flung open the door.

You know what? I kind of love this ending. Yes, I could have got *that* ending. But this one was perfect in its own way. Nothing too much. Nothing that made it awkward. Just enough to feel the swell of my heart. In that moment I felt whole.

I know Paddy took me to the debs because he was kind and because I asked. I know he said yes because he could tell what it would mean to me. I knew even then that he didn't have romantic feelings for me. He was older, living in London, I wasn't naïve. But I was a young girl who needed a date to her debs, and he came through and played the part to a T.

During the night he gave me his bow tie, an Abbeyleix tradition. I think I still have it. A memento of the other thing Paddy gave me – something I have cherished my whole life. The experience of romance. And for someone like me, it meant the world.

Mom sometimes says I should date, even now. When I was a bit younger, she'd ask if I'd ever think about going out with someone else who had EB, and I'd always give her the same answer: 'Why would I? I already have it.'

It's just the truth.

Because the truth is, I never wanted to date someone with a disability – not because I don't respect it, but because I didn't want *that* to be the reason we were together.

I didn't want someone to see me as part of a category. I want to be seen as a person.

As Emma.

That's what the debs gave me. That's why the memory of that night is etched in me so deeply.

For one night, I felt like a woman.

Not a patient. Not a cause. A woman in a beautiful dress on the arm of a kind boy, slow dancing.

It was perfect.

No kiss?

Even better.

That's a great ending.

14

You're on Your Own, Kid

College was going to be my chance to start fresh, to be just Emma. No footnotes, no history. I'd spent years being whispered about, pushed aside, mocked and pitied in secondary school. College would be different, and I knew exactly where I wanted to go for my next chapter. The Limerick Institute of Technology.

Both of my parents are from Limerick, and we'd spent so many weekends there that it felt like a second home. I knew the place, I loved the city. It made sense that that's where I'd begin again.

I wanted to study business and marketing. It was a practical move: business would be something that opened doors but didn't box me in, and marketing was interesting. I studied and hoped for the points to get a place on the course.

College wasn't just going to be a new subject – it was a new life. I'd be living away from home for the first time. I would be independent. Doing my own thing, deciding my own schedule. There'd be Freshers' Week, Rag Week, pub crawls, nights out and new people. I imagined myself drifting from lecture halls to student cafés, making friends and going to parties, living the kind of life I'd seen on telly.

After my Leaving Cert, Mom and I went back to Lourdes.

We didn't go for any particular reason, we just took up the offer of a spot and went.

On our last day we were in the grotto and Mom whispered, 'Emma, ask Our Lady for something you need,' in the lowest voice she could manage. She reached out and touched the wall of the grotto. I looked around. My mother's eyes were closed. It all felt really serious.

I knew immediately what I should ask for. My constant throat operations were becoming unbearable. I'd have to go into hospital for three or four days every few months and suffer, yet nothing was improving. I'd be good for a month max, then regress to choking a few times a day.

I'd never really thought about asking for help like this in Lourdes. I had faith, but here I was putting my faith *into* something, pressing my hand to the wall with my mother, asking Our Lady from the bottom of my heart to heal my throat. It was an expression of belief, not in this one God or this particular saint, but in something bigger than me. I made my prayer with the cold wall under my palm. Mom prayed too.

Then we forgot about it.

When we got back, I applied for one of those on-campus share houses – the ones with a good few bedrooms, shared kitchen, students coming and going. I got my results, the points I needed, and I was lucky enough to be offered the course I wanted. So I was all set. Limerick was to be my new home. It felt like a real slice of independence.

College was a massive shift for Mom. For eighteen years she'd cared for me every single day – acted as my shepherd as well as mothering me, changing my dressings, soothing my wounds, coaxing me when I wouldn't eat. Now she had to let me go.

But look, we are Fogartys. New things are always on the cards and so, in good spirits, Catherine helped me sort my suitcase while Mom and Dad packed the car. We headed down the day before term started, boot full of duvets and jackets, a kettle, a box of bandages, medication and creams. We were nervous, but we all wanted this for me, without a doubt.

When we pulled up at the house we were met by the man managing the accommodation. He was smiling and he shook Dad's hand, but as he greeted us his voice took on this strange sheepish tone. It turned out I was the only person moving in. Nobody else in the whole college had ticked the box on the form that said they'd be happy to share a house with someone disabled.

Not *one* person.

That little square on the form became a wall between me and the 'normal' student experience I was craving.

'Are you kidding me?' I said. I meant it to break the tension, but my voice caught a bit at the end.

The man looked embarrassed. 'You can still live here, Emma, of course. You can have the whole house for the price of a single room.'

To him, that was a great deal. More space probably would be a dream for most people. But I hadn't wanted space. I'd wanted *people*.

I know that checkbox hadn't said, 'Do you want to avoid Emma Fogarty?' But in my head, it may as well have.

'You'll be able to have friends over at least,' Dad offered, trying to soften the blow. 'Plenty of room for visitors.'

But I could see it in his face. He was upset too. This wasn't what any of us had pictured.

I'd believed college would be different. I thought students

would be open-minded, mature and kinder. But on the very first day, I got the same message I'd been getting since first year in secondary school. *You're not one of us.*

That caused something to crumble a little in me. A little fall under the surface. I thought, *I'm eighteen. I'm still here. But people don't want to be friends with me.*

Mom cried in the kitchen of the accommodation when she thought I wasn't looking.

Poor Mom. And poor Dad. Letting go of me after a lifetime of care wasn't easy. And it was made even harder knowing I was stepping into a world that had already rejected me, quietly, with the absence of a tick of a pen on a form. I told them I'd be fine and I'd come home at weekends. I told them I wanted to do this.

After a really emotional farewell, where we were all feeling it, my family left to drive back home and I was left alone.

That first night, I slept on my own in a house for the first time in my life. Every sound felt amplified – creaks, taps, the fridge humming. I lay in bed in the dark and whispered to myself, over and over, 'You'll be fine, Emma. You'll be fine. You'll be fine.'

By morning, I almost believed it. I decided that, even like this, I'd make my college dream come true. I'd study. I'd go out. I'd prove to every single checkbox-unticked student that I didn't need them. I could do this on my own.

But Mom couldn't rest.

'What if you fall?' she said on the phone. 'What if something happens?'

So she arranged for a woman, Mary, an old school friend of hers who lived nearby, to pop in every day to check I was still in one piece.

'She will stay some nights too,' Mom told me.

I didn't love the idea – part of me was clinging to the belief that I could look after myself – but I understood. I let Mom organise it. She needed that more than I did.

* * *

I started college in earnest, introduced myself to my lecturers, explained my condition and warned them about my choking. One of the first lecturers I met knew about EB, so I didn't have to explain the whole thing.

I'd had a throat operation during the summer, but the relief only ever lasted three months max. On my first week I had already run out of time and could feel the usual sensation of choking in my throat. I was going to have to go back for more surgery. I knew it and I was dreading it.

About a month in, a new lecturer started. After class I went up to introduce myself, tell him about my disability and explain that I often struggle with my condition.

'Sometimes I might even have to leave because I ch–' I said, then stopped talking. Something had just hit me.

'That's no problem,' he said, 'if you need to leave that is fine ...'

But I was miles away. I turned and left the class and rang Mom straight away.

'Mom, I haven't choked once in a month,' I said, 'not since about a week after I started college.'

My mother was blown away.

'Let's not speak too soon,' she said, 'but I really hope you got your miracle, Emma.'

I did get it. I rarely choked again for another twenty years. Suddenly I could eat most things, even chicken wings or potato waffles. I became absolutely obsessed with something Mom made, where she would fry small chunks of boiled potato and thin slices of onion together until they were soft. I could not get enough of it. I tried things I'd never eaten before – anything potato was a win for me. I stuffed my face with chocolate and soft cakes. I was still careful, but the regular bouts of choking became a thing of the past.

What made it even more magic was that everyone was so delighted to see it! My parents, my family, my doctors. I was still getting my main nutrition through the tube at night, but in the day I was snacking like there was no tomorrow and putting on weight. I was so healthy.

I don't know what it was – a higher power, a Holy Ghost, or just my body listening to me – but something changed on that trip to Lourdes.

Because of it I *believe* in miracles.

* * *

College was the first time I started working with the Centre for Independent Living, which is a government-funded group that provides personal assistance to people who have limited mobility or a disability. For me it was life-changing, and it gave me real freedom, where before I had to rely on my mom. I love my mother and I really love her company. But at nineteen I wanted freedom as a young college student on my own and the Centre for Independent Living gave me a sense of that.

The relationship is not so much carer and patient, as personal assistant and leader. That is how we refer to our roles and how it works best. The personal assistant comes with me where *I* want to go and assists me with little things I can't do for myself. This gives me independence and normalcy. It balances the playing field and gives me freedom from relying on favours from those I love to help me do the things I want to do. It also gives freedom back to those people who love me enough to spend their time doing them.

The Centre for Independent Living trains the PAs who are going to work with EB patients. First, they get a general overview of what EB is and how it affects someone. After that they get hands-on training with nurses, shadowing real bandage-changes and learning the daily routines – how to do the bandages themselves, how to spot trouble areas on the skin, how to help without hurting the person. It's not easy work and they're not nurses, but they need to be capable. The centre is funded by the government, so there's always a balance of bureaucracy and humanity at play.

Having a PA is a massive part of life with EB. It's personal, intimate work. And you don't get to choose who you work with. You're not part of the decision-making process of who it is that you will be spending so much time with every week. So when it's a good fit, when you work well with the person, it's a gift.

When it's not and you don't, it's really exhausting. I've experienced both.

One of my first PAs was Laura. I loved her so much, right from the get-go. She was a nurse in training, so helping me with bandages was nothing to her. She was great at doing them. We weren't too different in age: she was twenty-one and I was nineteen. I remember she invited me to her twenty-first birthday celebrations and I had a brilliant time. I got myself a pair of pink, heeled boots in Penneys. They had a wedge heel of only about an inch, but of course a night of dancing around in cheap shoes is good for no one, let alone someone with EB with a weakness in their foot bones. By the time the party was over and we were walking back to her house, I was really feeling the pain, but I didn't want to complain. Laura's friends were so fun and I was having a ball.

'How far is it?' I said at one point on the journey, coming to a complete stop. Typical of EB to get in my way.

'Just up the top of this hill,' Laura told me.

'I don't think I can get up there,' I admitted. I remember she looked at me, then turned around and started backing up to me, before bending over. She looked at me from under her hair. 'Get on my back,' she said.

Look, we'd all had a few drinks, me included, so I got up on her back and she carried me the rest of the way. I suppose the giddiness of the adventure I was having stopped me from feeling the pain of her hip bones digging into my thighs, but by the time I started feeling it we were standing in her bedroom and I was soaked in blood. I hid in there once I realised, but her friend saw me upset and told Laura. She sought me out.

'Are you wounded?' she said, her head coming around the door.

It was bad.

'Right,' Laura said, 'have you bandages with you?'

I nodded, slowly. I could not believe how kind Laura was.

Then and there, on her twenty-first birthday night, Laura abandoned her friends and her after-party and spent an hour in the room with me doing my bandages.

I have never forgotten that.

I'm still in touch with Laura and she even named her second daughter Frankie Emma Hession, which just shows how much she cares about me.

15

You Are Not Alone

Within a few months of starting college, I had got to know a few girls from my course. They were really nice, quiet girls from all over the country and we sat together most days. Then one day I overheard someone say there was a house party happening that weekend. We were sitting in a group, but I was slightly on the outside of it.

'We should all go,' one of the girls said.

I waited for the lull, the silent exchange of eyes. I waited for them to whisper that they should talk about it later. I waited to be hurt.

But it didn't happen.

She turned right around and asked me, 'Have you something to wear?'

'I might go to Penneys,' another girl said, 'see what they have.'

I nodded along, but I felt like I was on fire with the excitement. I was invited.

I went home, rooted through my wardrobe, and picked out the outfit I thought looked the most effortless and cool – you know the way you want to look like you didn't try too hard, even though you've tried on seven different tops already.

On the day of the party I did my hair and make-up. I was

so excited. But then I hit a moment where this independence wasn't exactly working for me. I had nobody to help me close buttons or do zips.

Sugar.

At home I had Mom, Dad and Catherine who would zip me up, close jeans or jackets as routine. Although I had Mary, my mom's friend, come in in the mornings to do the same, now I was standing in this empty house with no way to get dressed in the clothes I wanted to wear. And the clock was ticking.

Like an angel sent from heaven, Mary chose that moment to call in.

'Mary! Mary!' I said. 'I'm supposed to meet my friends, can you do up these jeans?'

Mary obliged.

'Where are you going?' she said and I told her all about the party.

'Right,' she said, 'you go and enjoy yourself, and I'll wait up for you and help you get out of that outfit.'

Thank God for Mary.

The party was *exactly* like you'd imagine it – paper cups, loud music, half the year packed into a terrace house with open doors and spill-outs onto the street. Lads messing. Couples leaning on kitchen counters, sitting on stairs, dancing in the tiny sitting room. Tables covered in cans and crisps and ashtrays. Someone already passed out in the hall. That quintessential lovely mess of Irish youth.

I had a few drinks. Not too much, just enough to feel like I was in it – not watching from the outside. And I went home unscathed.

Nobody stared. Nobody whispered.

And for that one night, I felt like a typical college student.

Not the girl with EB. Not the girl who lives alone. Not the disability people didn't tick the box for.

Just me.

* * *

College was meant to be the start of everything real, and, in some ways, it was. I had my friends in class, though they went home most weekends. But I was out in the world, on my own, doing my thing – walking to lectures, getting through bandage changes on my own terms, making myself a cup of tea in a quiet kitchen before 9 a.m. I could never take notes, but the lecturers would usually make a copy of their own notes and I could study from that. It wasn't easy, but I can honestly say I did my best. I read and read till the cows came home.

After a few weeks, I got a call from the man who ran the student housing.

'There are a few girls looking for a swap,' he said. 'Not getting on with their current housemates. I mentioned your place has a couple of rooms free. They're eager.'

I said yes straight away, no question. I wanted what everyone else had – people to chat to in the kitchen, the clatter of someone making tea while you finish a late-night essay.

So, a few days later, Emer and Joanne moved in.

And things were good at the start. The kitchen was busy. We made meals. We shared. There was laughter, casual chats, good-natured moaning about assignments. I was really excited. This was the college life I had dreamed of.

* * *

One random day around the time the girls moved in, I went to see the disability liaison officer. I wanted to get a handle on what kind of supports were available, and she was great – warm and helpful – running through the various things they could do for me. She mentioned that she would put me in touch with a local guy who knew everything there was to know about voice recognition technology. He was the fastest in Ireland at using it, at that time. The liaison officer thought I should try the tech for myself.

'Here is his number,' she said, handing me a piece of paper with a name and telephone number on it. 'He will be able to run through the whole thing with you and …'

Her voice faded away because I was staring at the paper.

I read it. Robert O'Neill.

And my brain stopped.

'Wait,' I said, interrupting. 'Do you mean Robert O'Neill, as in *Bobby* O'Neill?'

She looked confused. 'I only know him as Robert.'

But I knew him as Bobby. Of course I knew him. It *was* Bobby. Bobby O'Neill from the EB clinics, the boy on the path ahead. He had always been in my life, but I'd never really known him – not properly. What were the chances? It was mad, really.

I texted him straight away.

Bobby called around to the house that same week, just to say hi. Because of my new roommates we didn't have anywhere private to sit but my bedroom, so that's where we ended up. It was awkward at first, both of us perched there at opposite ends of the bed. At first we were both waiting for the other to say something, but then – God knows who went first – once the talking started, it didn't stop.

Bobby was kind and instantly loyal. He was so funny too.

He loved driving and he loved pool – a sport he could manage with EB. He was a superfan of Michael Jackson. We texted constantly, all day, into the small hours of the morning. We weren't the phone-call type. Bobby's texts became a little thread that ran through everything I was going through. I had a real friend on the other end of the line who didn't need back story. He knew the pain, the routines, the stares, because he dealt with it all too. We had similar issues and the same form of EB.

'My left foot is my weak zone,' he told me.

'Stop,' I said, 'me too!'

Our friendship made everything feel a bit easier. Suddenly, we both had someone in our life who got it. Someone who *knew* what EB felt like.

Bobby and I were both doing something the other wanted. I was living independently. He wanted to move out. He was driving. I wanted to learn. Just knowing the other was managing and living gave us hope. Like, if you can do it, maybe I can too. Bobby had a great way of thinking about life.

'*Carpe diem*,' he would say, 'seize the day.'

We never dated. There are still people who refuse to believe that because we were so close, but we never did. It would have been too much, I think. I can think of nothing harder than loving someone who suffers like you do. There would be nothing sadder than watching each other decline. It wouldn't have worked. Instead, he was my best friend.

* * *

One night, after we had been living together a few months, I was heading to bed when Emer and Joanne stopped me in the hall.

'We were just wondering,' they said, with wide eyes and smiles, 'what Laura does in the room with you?'

I blinked.

What did Laura *do*? It seemed like such a strange question.

'She helps me,' I said. I knew they knew that already. They could see my bandages. They could see my wounds. They'd watch me limp around the house with bone ache. They knew I couldn't eat popcorn and crisps like they could. What did they think Laura was doing? Playing Monopoly?

Then they cornered Laura too, asking her straight out. She didn't answer.

'They were asking me what I'm doing in the room with you,' Laura told me after. 'Sure don't they *see* your bandages? They know full well what I'm helping with. So I didn't bother answering them.'

That should have been the end of it.

But it wasn't.

There were sly looks and whispers. Things I recognised from school, a sort of quiet around their hellos and goodbyes. A long pause before replying to me. No chat any more. If I asked how they were, they would blankly smile and repeat the same old, 'Fine, how are you?' Then they would immediately leave.

'Emma,' Emer said one day, 'can you do the hoovering today?'

I stared at her. Over my last few years in school, from all the writing, blisters on the insides of my fingers had turned to scars, and the scars pulled my fingers in. I had really limited use of my hands because of that. I hadn't lost the use of them fully yet, but it wasn't long away. People with my form of EB often find that scar tissue forces our fingers together and fuses them. Our fingers become encased in these sort of mittens of scar tissue. Still in there and still technically working but no good to us at all.

Emer could see how my hands were, but still I was forced to say, 'Oh, I can't hold the hoover.' It made me feel awful. I said, 'I'll ask Laura, if you want.'

She said, 'Grand, if you wouldn't mind,' and walked off.

The next day: same thing.

It kept happening. Over and over.

And I thought, *I've done this before. I've been in this corridor. I've been on this bus. I know this script.*

Eventually, I snapped.

'Stop asking me to hoover,' I said. 'You *know* I can't hold it.'

They looked at each other. Then Joanne said it.

'It's just that ...' and she looked at Emer, not at me. 'It's just that we don't want to be hoovering up the flakes of your skin. It freaks us out.'

I didn't respond.

I couldn't.

I was too embarrassed, too shocked. Yes, my skin sometimes flakes – mostly from my hands where the scar tissue gets dry. This is part of my disability.

It's not like I was leaving trails behind me like some kind of human dandruff machine. God.

The tension in the house became thick. I'd walk into a room and my roommates would leave. No matter what. They'd get up one after the other, even if they were mid-conversation or mid-meal, and walk out. No words, no explanations. Just up and out.

Thank God for Laura. I told her everything.

'Feck them, Emma,' she'd say, 'they're looking for something. They'd want to watch it.'

And she meant it. Laura gave me care, but she also gave me courage.

Then, one night, I went to knock on their door to ask them to open a bottle for me. That was all.

They opened the door. I asked. Emer snatched the bottle, twisted the cap, shoved it back into my hand and shut the door in my face.

I thought about it for days after.

At first, I felt guilty. At first, I tried to find reasons that two girls would be so mean. I thought back over everything that had happened up to that point. I didn't know if they'd just decided they didn't like me any more, or maybe they'd listened at the door and overheard me complaining to Laura about their silent treatment, because I had been. Maybe I'd caused this.

At that point I was so low, really believing that I was the problem. I didn't even give EB any of the credit, I just blamed *me* and told myself I would never have friends, I would always be an outcast.

Laura was having none of that.

'They're looking for something to gossip over,' she would say again and again, and it would ease my heart a little. I realised if they were listening, that was on them. And if they turned on me for no reason, that was on them too. And if the problem was that my skin was on the floor in tiny specks, well that was on them a hundredfold.

Because Laura was right. This was nothing to do with me. This was two bored girls bonding over the thrill of ganging up on someone vulnerable. Good for them.

But even though I knew they were the ones at fault, I still had to finish the year, once again, being isolated.

And I was suffering enough already.

Thankfully things were going to change forever. I just didn't know it yet.

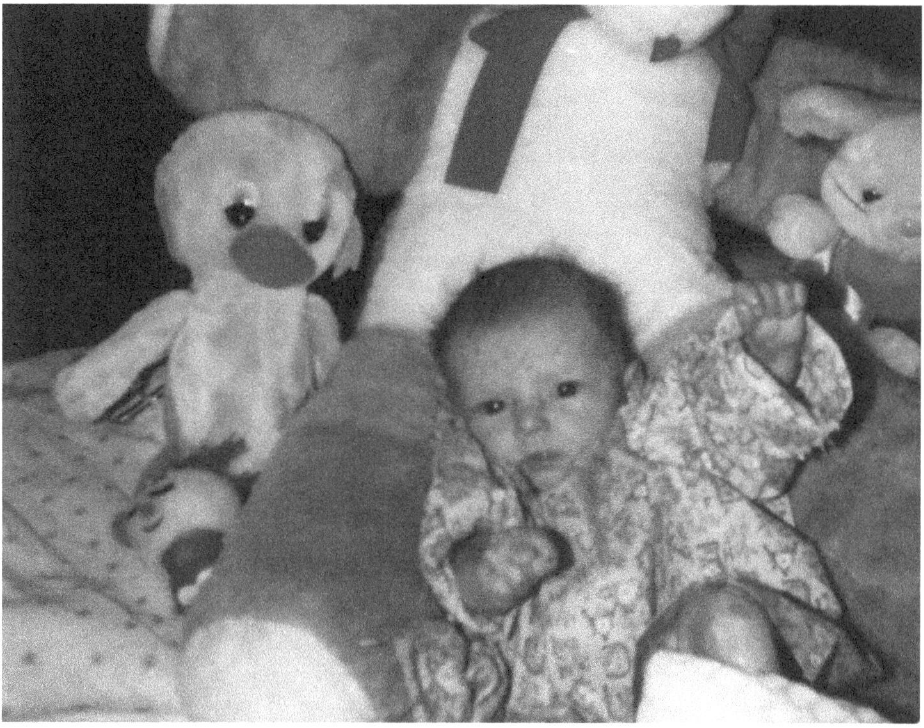

One of the first pictures of me at home, taken on 26 September 1984, in a dress that was sewn with the seams on the outside for me by one of the Bowens.

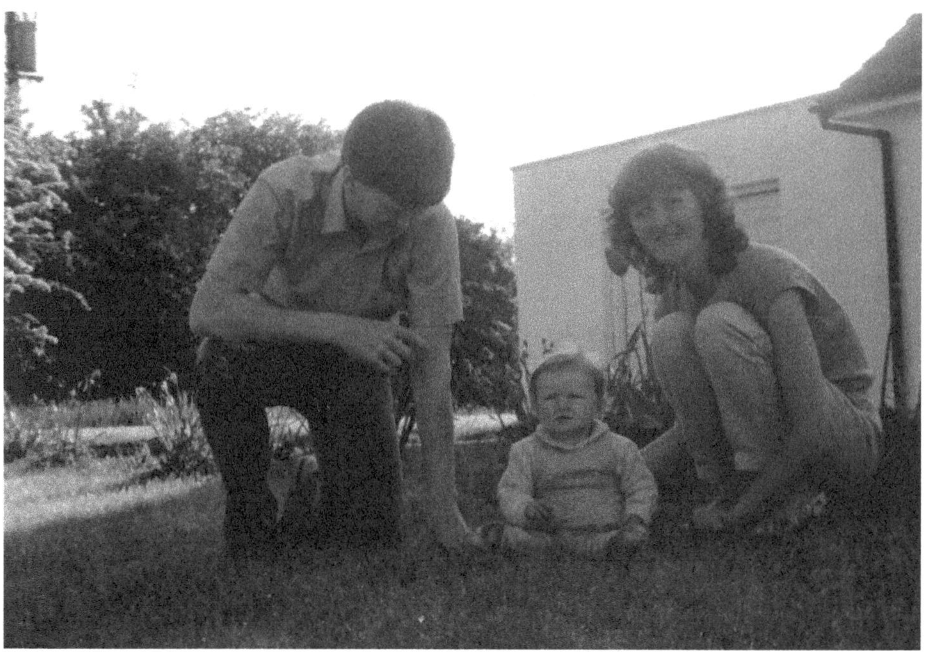

Mom, Dad and me in the garden of our Abbeyleix home on 7 June 1985.

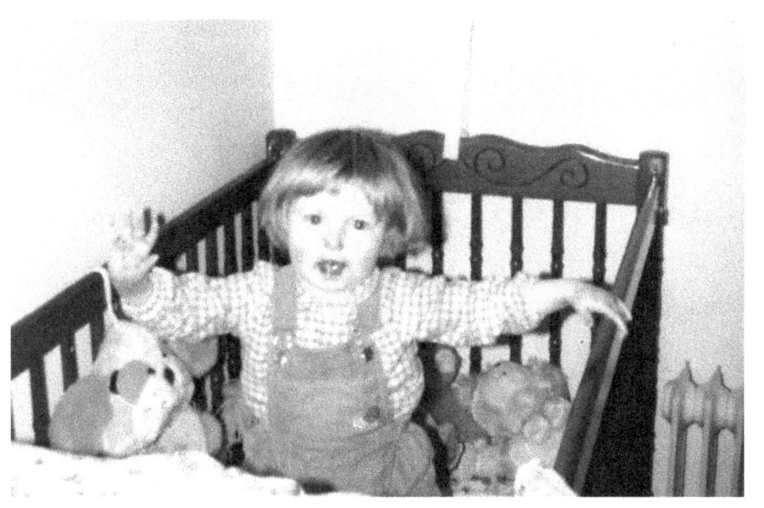
Me aged two.

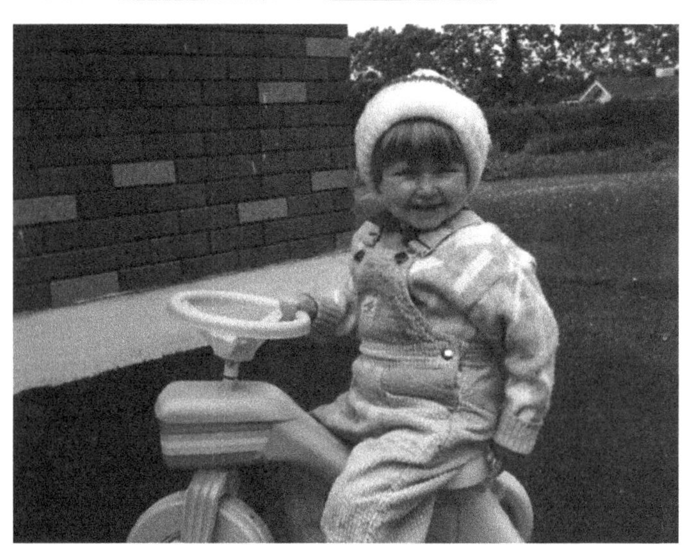
My first set of wheels, 25 June 1987.

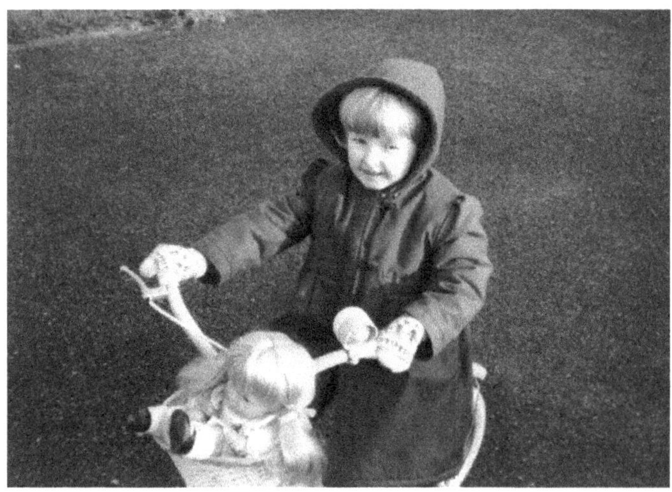
On my one and only bicycle, which was one of my most treasured possessions for the feeling of independence it gave me.

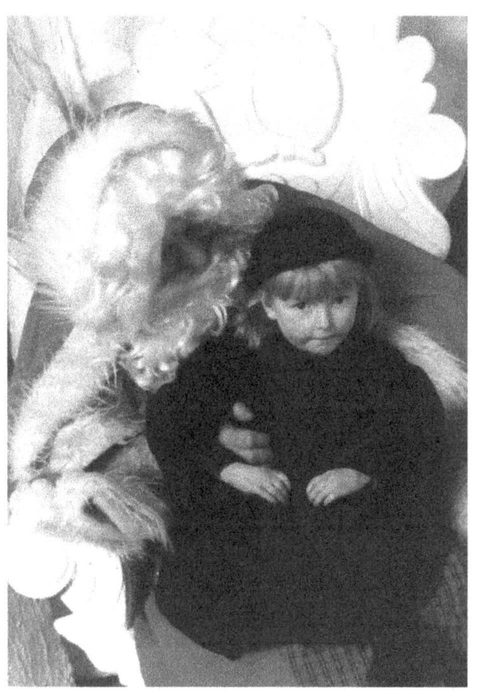

Christmas is one of my favourite times of year. It was Santa who brought me my bicycle.

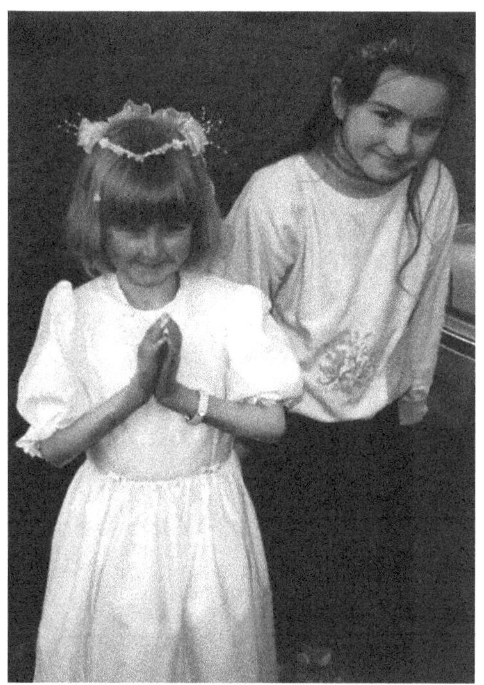

With my cousin Aoife on the day of my First Communion.

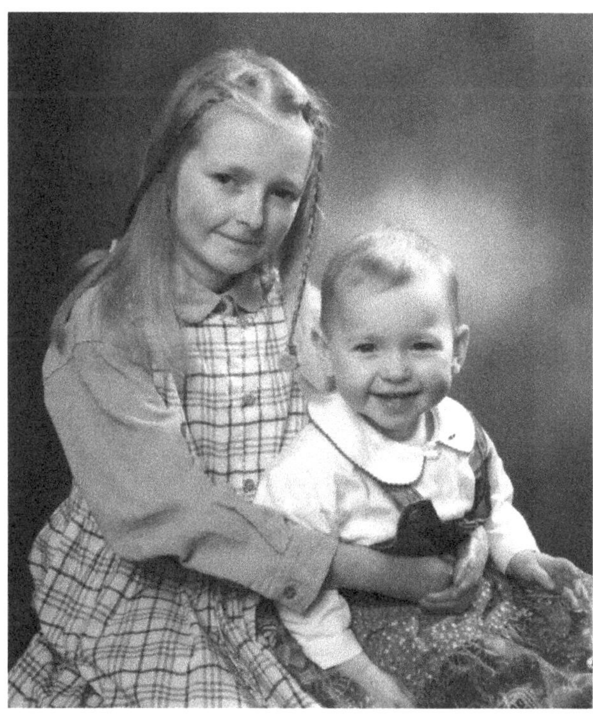

Me and Catherine, when she was one year old.

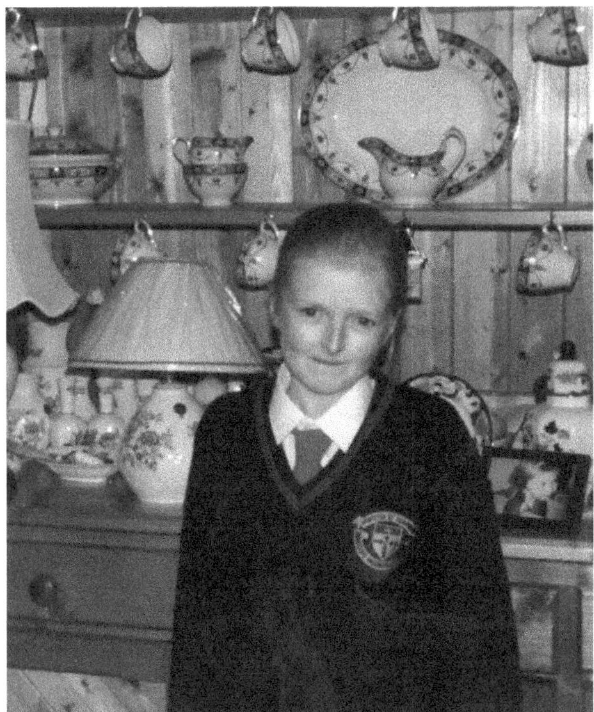

Ready for secondary school. While I had loved primary school, secondary school was not a happy experience for me.

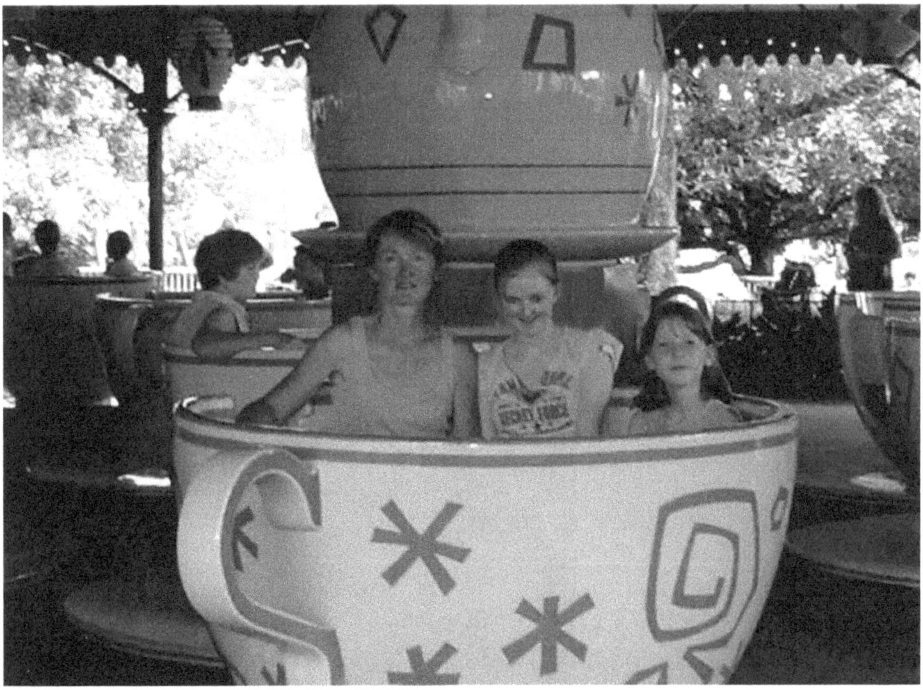

My favourite ride at Disneyland, Florida, was the Tea Cups. I loved spinning around, as you can probably guess from the big grin on my face.

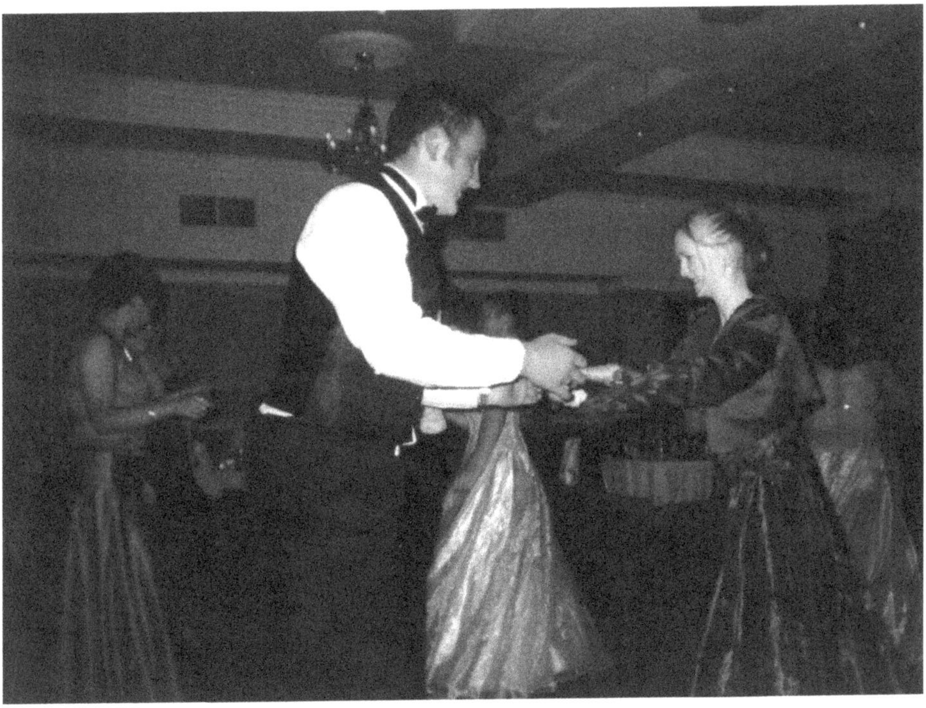

At my debs with Paddy Moran, who was the perfect date and even persuaded me to dance. It was a night I'll never forget.

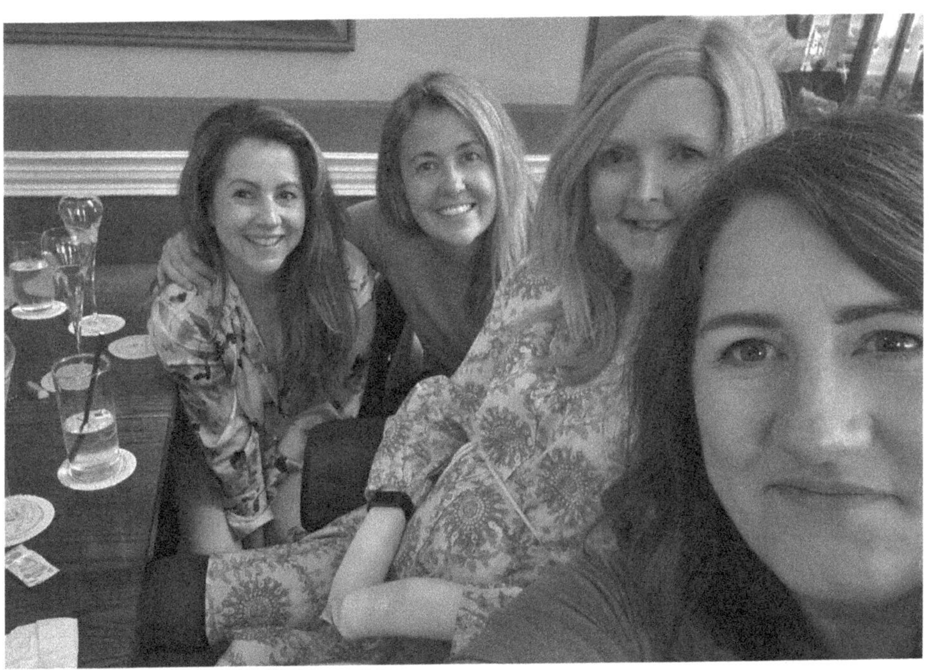

Me and the girls – Kim, Lynn and Caitriona – the best friends a girl could have, we have so much fun together.

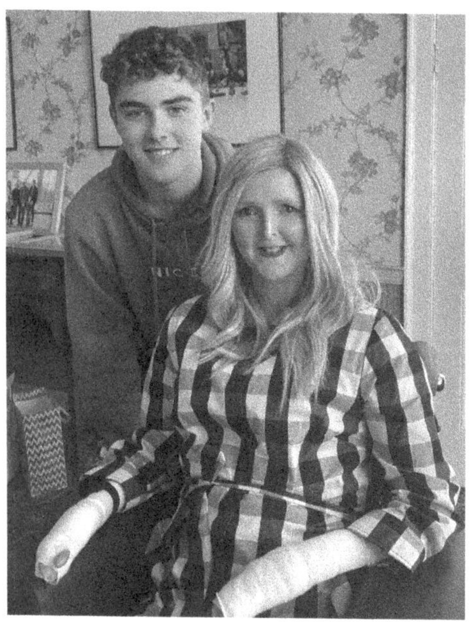

With my amazing godson, Sean. I'm so proud to be his godmother.

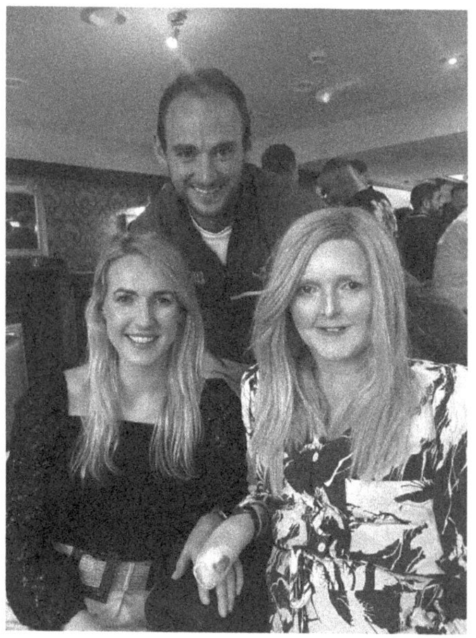

With Catherine and her lovely boyfriend, Tiernan. I couldn't have asked for a better sister.

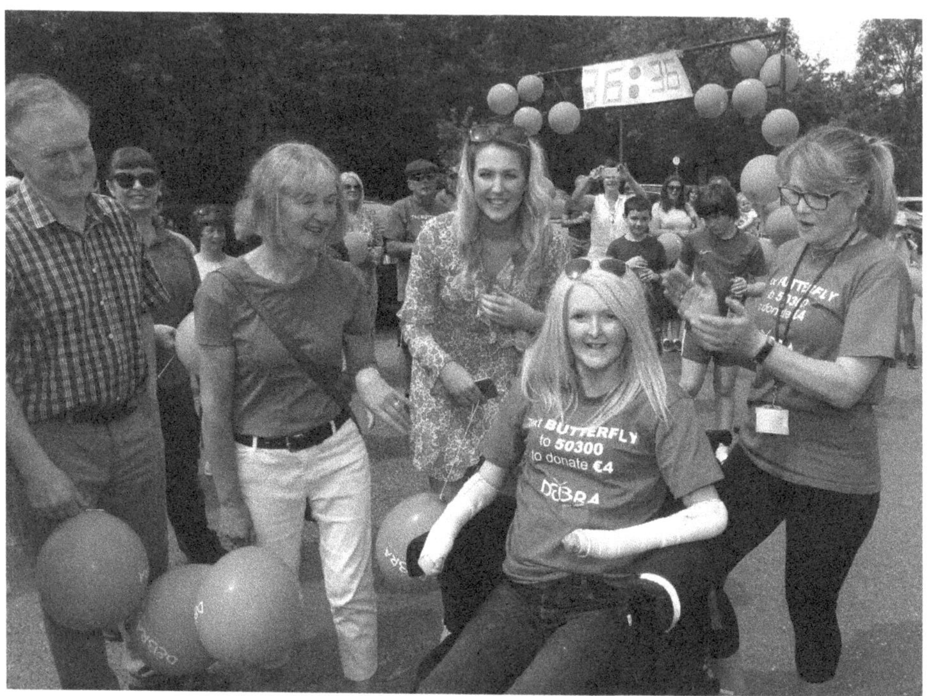

Celebrating at the end of Emma's 36 Challenge with Dad, Mom, Catherine and George. George and I became known as 'the girls in blue' during our walks. My cousin Nicola is behind us in green.

I have been so lucky to have the support of the O'Gorman family over the years, I don't know what I'd have done without them.

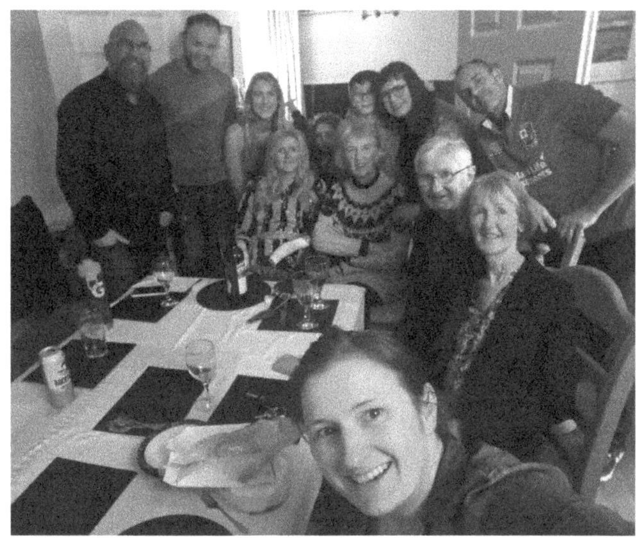

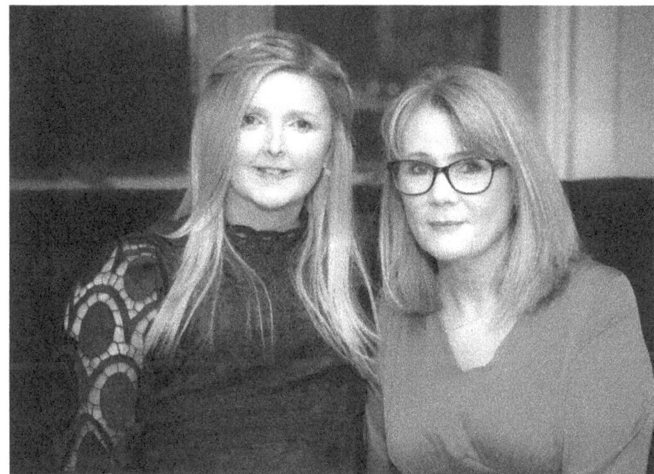

At my fortieth birthday party with George, who is so much more to me than my full-time PA – we are true friends. © Richard Sheehy / www.richardsheehy photography.com

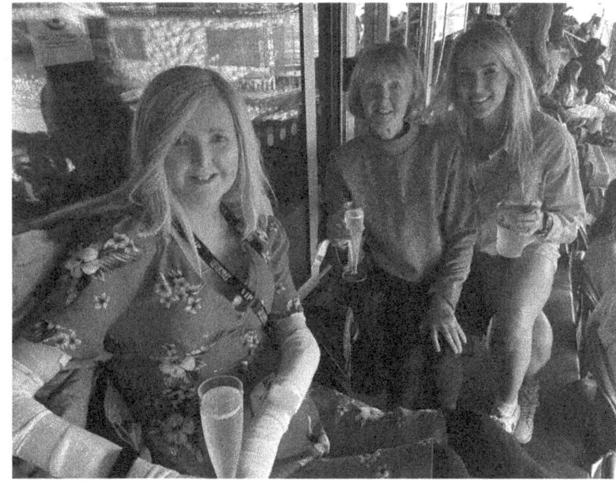

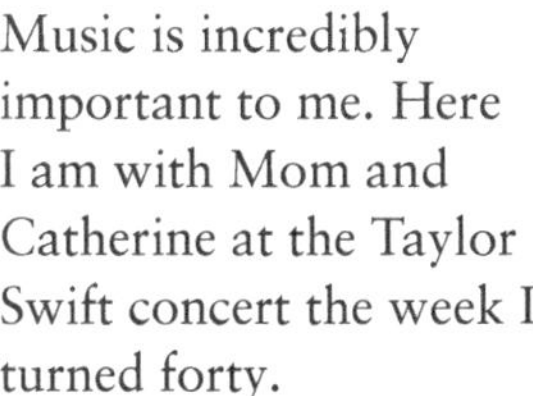

Music is incredibly important to me. Here I am with Mom and Catherine at the Taylor Swift concert the week I turned forty.

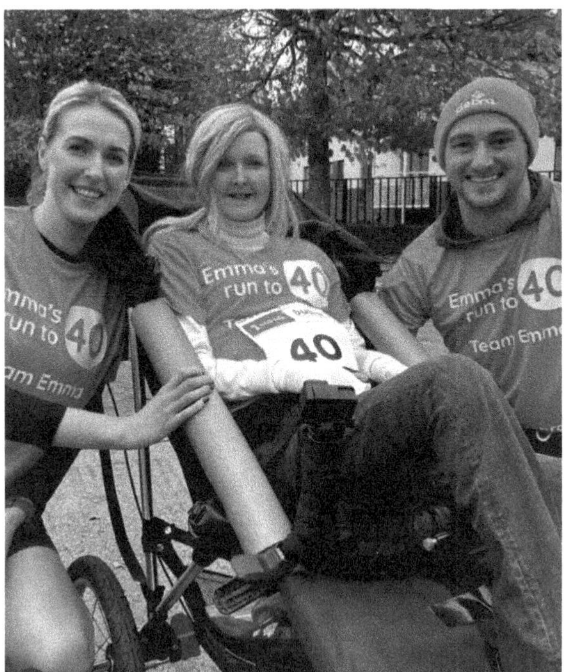

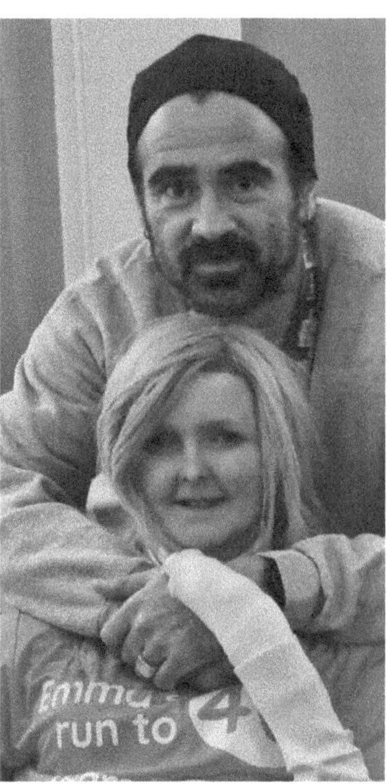

The Dublin Marathon was the most amazing day for me. Colin Farrell ran the whole marathon to help me raise money for Debra Ireland and pushed me the last four kilometres, one for each decade of my life, with Catherine and Tiernan running alongside us.

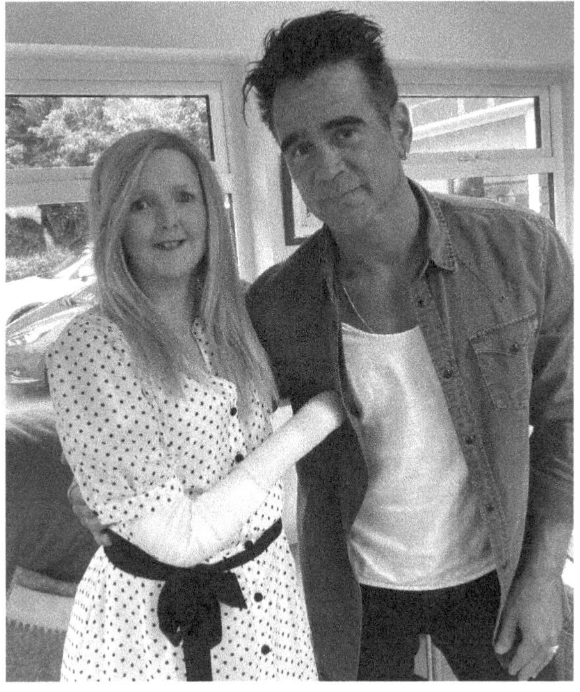

Colin has been the most wonderful friend over the years.

Part Two

Being Emma

16

Firework

I feel like I have grown up with Debra Ireland. It never felt like a charity to me, more like something I was deeply connected with, a community, a purpose. And Debra gave a shape to my life at a time when I really needed that.

It all came about towards the end of that first year of college.

Despite feeling low and isolated again, I was involved in a television event with Debra Ireland, talking about my life with EB as a way to highlight the condition and make it more known in a world where it was rare and largely unheard of. I wanted to do these things with Debra Ireland, because I wanted people to see EB. I wanted them to think, *Oh, so that's what that looks like.* Someone has to show the world that this rare thing is real for so many – this is not an idea, this is our real lives. EB has faces, names and families.

When I was doing the television interview, the presenter asked me what I was up to.

'I'm in college,' I said, 'in Limerick, studying business and marketing.'

I had never connected what I was doing for my degree with the charity that supported me, but those in Debra did. No sooner had we gone off air, than my phone rang.

It was Mom.

'Emma, the CEO of Debra just called me,' she said. 'She didn't know you were studying business and she asked if there was any help they could give you.'

'That's amazing,' I said, and joked, 'Can they give me a summer job?'

'I asked the same thing,' Mom said, 'and she said, of course.'

I was delighted.

'That's you sorted now,' Dad said.

I had, to that point, only seen Debra Ireland when they were outside, doing things. I didn't see what went on behind closed doors. Debra is a charity, yes – but it's also a business. That might sound blunt, but it's the truth. People think of charities as these soft, well-meaning little things, all bake sales and ribbons. But no. You have to run a charity the way you'd run a company – clear-eyed and accountable. You have to be tight with the purse strings and sharper still with the mission. Because people give their money, but they also give you their trust, and they deserve to have both of those things treated with respect.

Debra has a board and it's made up of half patrons and half businesspeople. That's not by accident. It's a system carefully honed to make this charity work the best it can.

Because EB is important.

I worked three days a week in fundraising in the summer. That's where I met Clyde, Anne and most of the people who would become my closest friends. I was the only one in the office with EB, but I never felt like the odd one out. That place gave me belonging. It gave me purpose. Clyde became like a big brother to me, he is one of those solid good guys, a real friend to all.

One day I was telling him that I used to ride horses as a child, and we talked about horses and how lovely they were.

Then, a few weeks later when I saw him, he said, 'Emma, do you want to come to the Horse Show with me and my fiancée at the weekend?'

I said yes, of course, and it was lovely. I got to know Clyde and Abigail, his now wife, so well. I even got to know Abigail's parents, and whenever there were events or dos on, I would stay with them. I'd wake up in the morning to tea and toast, and I loved spending time there.

Clyde was good to me, always keeping an eye on me. One night he got me into a concert he was working at. Girls Aloud were on stage and he walked with me down to see if we could meet them coming off stage. I didn't know him very well then, and so I didn't want to be rude and tell him I was struggling with the ground and the distance. It was so warm that day, not a cloud in the sky. I didn't want to make a fuss, since he was being so good. So I kept going.

'I think it's around here,' Clyde said and looked across at me just as I was starting to wobble. He noticed me go suddenly pale, sprang into action and got me water and shade straight away.

Little moments like that made me really trust him, and so he became one of my best friends.

That summer job was the beginning of a new place for me, and the beginning of a better experience.

I'll never forget the first time I walked into the Debra Ireland office. Because of how they ran things, because of the events they had and the amazing organising that was clearly going on behind the scenes, I was expecting a fancy office laid out with desks and fancy phones and carpets.

I expected a front desk with a receptionist and busy phone lines jammed with charitable donations.

What I found was a bright little room in an unmarked building right on the edge of Dublin.

And you know what? It made me love my charity even more.

Because all that amazing work – the campaigns, the clinics, the community – it was all coming out of this tiny engine room, the work of a handful of people who really gave a damn.

* * *

In second year in college, I moved into a house with three other girls – Linda, Noreen and Sabrina.

I was on my guard, of course I was. But this felt different from the start. Maybe it was my summer spent working in Dublin, maybe I was just less tolerant and laying my cards out a little harder than before, but I had no trouble at all with these new housemates.

They were older than me and had that mature edge to them. We got on. They accepted my restrictions and accepted me as I was.

It felt … easy. They didn't sneak off for one-on-ones, they didn't whisper. There were no looks, no isolation. None of us paired up, we were all equal.

Everything felt like it had in my head when I thought of having roommates. And I don't mean that in a 'we all wore matching pyjamas and had pillow fights' kind of way. I mean it in the way you crave when your life has never really been ordinary.

And most Thursdays we'd go across the road for one drink at the pub.

There was something about that small ritual that made everything feel *normal*. I remember my mom rang one time, just as we were settling in to the snug in the little local by the house. I picked up quickly to say, 'I can't talk, Mom, I'm at the pub. Just out for the one with the girls.'

'The *pub*?' she said, as if I'd just told her I was off to join the circus.

I smiled so wide.

'Yep,' I said, 'just for one!'

I was also working as much as I could, whenever I could, with Debra. I was budgeting my money and making things work. It was a student's life, but it was *mine*.

'How are you getting along?' Deirdre, the EB family support worker asked me one day. She used to check in with all of us in person and, to be honest, calling her a 'support worker' feels too small for what she was to us. Deirdre had a background in psychology and supported us emotionally, but more than that, she became a good friend to us all.

I was beaming telling her how things were going.

'Wow, Emma,' she said, 'good for you.'

My confidence was growing in spades.

In fact, it was out of control.

Clyde was getting married to Abigail that summer. The wedding was in Italy.

'I want to go to Clyde's wedding,' I told my parents.

'But we have America booked,' my dad said, 'we can't do two holidays.'

'Well, I want to go to the wedding,' I said, and my parents started to hum and haw and look at calendars. I stopped them in their tracks and said, 'By myself.'

I'll never forget my mother's face.

'I'm going,' I said and went to my room to book a flight.

Mom had serious reservations, but I was convinced. I told

myself I was living alone in college and I was able to do this and, yes, the hotel and wedding were on a hill, but I would be grand. I just wanted to be there, it meant a lot to me.

Then I was chatting to my childhood nurse Ursula about it.

'I've always wanted to go to Italy,' she said, 'I'll go with you if you like.'

Once she heard that, Mom relaxed.

So, it was all go. I bought a beautiful, full-length, baby-blue dress that I loved, and booked into a hotel with a view near the wedding venue. And when the time came and I found myself walking alone into the airport to meet everyone, with my little flight bag, I felt like a proper adult. I loved it.

The gang was all there at the airport, and when Clyde saw me he said, 'Well I didn't want to believe you'd make it, until right now, this minute, seeing you here.'

'I don't think I believed it either,' I said with a huge smile. EB is so unpredictable and we both knew that.

The day before the wedding, everyone decided to visit the island of Capri. I went too. Getting on the ferry was easy enough, as it was very accessible and I could walk on, no issue. We spent the crossing chatting, oblivious to the problem that was about to arise.

We were all excited as the ferry neared the island, when suddenly it stopped. The crew began to open doors and we weren't sure what was happening, so we looked overboard. There, bobbing below us, was this little motorboat and a narrow gangway, more of a steep ladder really, connecting the two. The island was being serviced by tender boat. The ferry was not going into the port.

'There is no way I can get down that!' I said.

Clyde asked if I could stay on the ferry.

'No, no, *signore*,' the man said, 'this ferry is going straight back to Sorrento.'

'Oh ...'

What on earth would we do?

Clyde was there, with his brothers and Abigail, and Abigail said, 'It's a pity we don't have a wheelchair.'

I looked at her like she had gone crazy.

'We could hold it,' she explained, 'and lower it down.'

I was just about to insist that I would never do that, I would be too frightened, when Clyde said, 'That's perfect,' and ran off. He came back less than a minute later with a chair from the café.

'Sit in this, Emma,' he said.

I didn't refuse; I knew we had no choice. And that is how I ended up being lowered off the side of a ship onto a small boat in the Mediterranean Sea.

Clyde and his brothers were the ones doing it. When I say I screamed – I mean it. I think 'DON'T DROP ME' is still echoing around the rocks of that island. It's funny now, but it wasn't funny at the time. Not even a little bit. The one time I glanced down, all I could see was beautiful, clear blue ocean and I thought I was about to go for a swim for sure. Then I caught sight of Clyde's face. He looked like he was performing surgery. And fair enough – dropping me was not exactly an option. But there were a couple of moments where I was dangling in mid-air thinking, *Alright, God, here I come. Get a cloud ready for me. I'm on the way.*

Of course, the Carroll brothers didn't let me bump off one single thing. They moved me down inch by inch. And somehow, they got me down. I did that mad abseil four times that day – onto the tender boat, off the tender boat, and back again to the ferry later.

It was mental. But I'm so glad I did it. I'm so glad I was there on Capri. It was a lovely place, although there were a few moments where I thought I would have to stop – Italy has a lot of steps!

At one point Clyde disappeared and when we looked for him, he was nowhere to be seen. He turned up again a few minutes later, jogging back to us with a cold drink for me. I couldn't stop laughing, knowing that he was remembering the concert two years earlier.

'I'm grand,' I promised him, but I'll admit now I was feeling the heat.

'Do you want to go back?' he said, and I know he would have dropped everything to bring me back to the port where it was flatter and easier. But I insisted we go on because I wanted to experience it *all*.

I wouldn't have missed it for the world.

That's the thing. I do mad stuff like this because the alternative is missing out. I'd rather deal with the awkwardness, the stares, the risk, than sit something out and regret it.

I was scared on that chair getting lowered onto the tender. Really scared. But my friends made it work. They looked after me.

On the last abseil, back onto the ferry, as I neared the top – I was hanging on with my eyes closed – I heard Abigail and others shouting, 'No! The chair! The chair!'

I think I squealed, waiting to hit the water.

'No!' Abigail kept calling up, 'the CHAIR!!'

I knew what the problem was a second later as two Italian men – trying to help and not understanding the extent of the problem – grabbed me by both arms (*oh oh*) and absolutely reefed me onto the ferry. Thank God Clyde's brother was there to catch me as I came through the doors like a bullet.

And the wedding, of course, was absolutely gorgeous. I wore the blue dress I loved so much. The only thing I was missing was the perfect pair of earrings. I love earrings and, to this day, I've always wanted a dangly gold pair, but it's almost impossible to get clip-ons and, unfortunately, with my condition, I can't get my ears pierced. It's frustrating that such a normal part of most girls' lives remains so out of reach for me.

Despite that, I still felt like a princess. I had prosecco and limoncello and stayed up as late as everyone else.

It felt so good to just be part of it all, and by myself. No one told me to take it easy. Nobody sent me to bed. There were no limits. Just *freedom*.

* * *

On the afternoon of my twenty-first birthday I was having my hair done by a friend, before my party, down in the house. The entire family was in the house – cousins, aunties and uncles. The only ones missing were my cousin Shane and his wife, Bethan, as they had had a baby boy the day before. They'd called him Sean after Shane's dad.

'It's so lovely,' I said to Mom, 'Sean must be delighted.'

Just then Aoife ran in with the house phone.

'Shane is ringing for you,' she said. I took the phone thinking it was unusual, he would normally text happy birthday. I supposed it was my twenty-first and maybe he thought that deserved a call instead. I answered straight away.

'Hiya,' I said, and he said happy birthday, and I said congratulations, and we caught up a little. Then he paused.

'Emma,' Shane said, 'can I tell you something and ask you something?'

'Sure,' I said, but I started shaking. I don't know why – I just felt this sense of something big about to happen.

'Emma, we think you are an incredible person,' he said, 'we can think of nobody more qualified to be a mentor or an inspiration, and we want you to be Sean's godmother.'

I will never forget that. In the moment, I filled with pride and tears – I don't think they stopped all day.

'I can't believe I am a godmother,' I told Shane, 'I won't let you down.'

I have tried to be there for Sean as much as I can, though he lives in Wales. I take my role seriously and travelled over for his baptism, of course, and again for his First Communion. He is an amazing guy, an adult himself now, almost twenty-one. It has been one of the great joys of my life to be part of his.

* * *

In third year, Linda, Noreen, Sabrina and I got the house together again. Those girls were lovely – not just nice in that polite, surface way, but properly sound. They were the kind of gang who remembered you had lectures in the same building they did and walked with you. The kind who waited for you to get up before putting on the kettle. We'd sit around the kitchen table chatting about everything and nothing. They didn't make a big deal about the bandages. They didn't act like my PA coming in was a scandal. They just let me live.

We stayed friends for years after college, and that says a lot. Because college friends can be like that – fun and then gone. But not them. They stuck.

For my final year I moved again, into another house share.

This time it was two girls and two lads. It was fine. It wasn't magic, but it wasn't a disaster either.

However, there was one weird thing I had to deal with. One of the lads never spoke to or looked at me. I don't mean he was shy, or quiet, or that he just kept to himself. I mean he actively avoided acknowledging that I existed. He never said hello. Never asked me a question. He never even nodded if we passed on the stairs. It was surreal. If he was looking for something in the kitchen, he'd search every drawer, every shelf – ten minutes of rummaging – and even then, he wouldn't ask if I'd seen it. He'd just keep looking or wait for someone else he could ask to come in.

Weirder still, if a friend of mine came over he'd spring to life. 'Hi, I'm –!' He'd chat away like he was the nicest fella in the world. It was almost worse than the outright meanness I'd dealt with before. Because with that, at least I knew where I stood. At least it was clear. This was something else. This was absence. A refusal to *see* me.

Despite him, though, I lived my life. I made it work in that house. Because that's what you do. And in the small spaces between the heavy days, you find things that keep you going.

Bobby had a great knack for lifting me out of any slump I found myself in. I'd be home, feeling overwhelmed with college and life with EB, and the doorbell or my phone would buzz and Bobby would be there. Somehow he always seemed to know when I needed some relief from it all. Always at the right moment, he would flood my phone with jokes and texts, or with encouragement.

Those little things, they matter more than you think. Especially when you're low.

And I *was* low, sometimes. No getting around that. I was

still living full-time with EB. I was still spending *all* of my life in pain.

But even so – I kept showing up. I sat my exams. I got my assignments in. I took notes, studied them while lying flat in bed. I kept going. I had my twenty-first birthday with all my friends and family, and it was really special. I danced with my father, which is a girl's dream; certainly, it was always mine. It was a wonderful moment. And finally, graduation.

Although, I nearly didn't. I failed one of my final exams by three points. Can I just say any teacher who fails a four-year degree over three points is a terrible person, and, for me, I just think it was cruel. I'd waited so long for that moment. Not the gown or the scroll or the photos, but the feeling of being done. Of making it through.

'You'll have to repeat the module,' I was told.

My parents went to the Education Board again and pleaded my case for me.

'Three points?' my father argued. 'Emma has had a huge disadvantage here.'

The answer came swift and fast on any sort of dispensation – it was a no. My mother and father appealed and appealed and appealed. They got letters from Debra to acknowledge my work there. They wanted the exams reviewed. They were, frankly, not taking no for an answer.

Eventually the Education Board allowed it, but they sent a letter to say that it was purely because of the work I was doing in my chosen field with Debra that they would allow three points to be added.

So I got my scroll.

Mom and Dad came down. Of course they did. They wouldn't have missed it for the world, but we didn't make a big fuss, as it had a sour tinge to it now. I don't think I even threw my hat up. I just showed up, lined up, collected my degree and walked back out again.

That was it.

I remember sitting at the dinner table that evening celebrating with Mom and Dad, the scroll resting on my lap. We had dinner out in a lovely place in Bunratty, and a little glass of prosecco. Nothing fancy. But it felt like a feast.

'You did it,' Mom said.

'I did,' I said. I didn't cry. But I felt everything then, in that moment, and I did feel my accomplishment, no matter what the college had done or said. Because behind that piece of paper was every morning I'd woken up in pain and still made it to class. It was every night I'd sat on my bed with raw wounds and still opened the books. It was every awkward moment in the kitchen, every cold shoulder, every room where someone walked out on me.

Behind that degree was *me*. It was every version of me that kept going, even when I didn't want to.

I was ready for the world then. Or at least, I thought I was.

I didn't know yet how the world would respond – how tough it would get, how buildings would shut me out, how many forms I'd have to fill in just to be allowed to live.

I didn't need a big hurrah. I didn't need confetti or a grand gesture. I didn't even need this paper if I was honest.

What I had was enough.

I was done.

I had survived college.

I was ready for whatever came next.

Little did I know, it would be *everything*.

17

Part of Your World

I took a year off after college. I spent most of it in a wheelchair. I was exhausted. Four years of full-time study while dealing with my illness had taken its toll and I was also suffering with my left foot again. Badly.

My hands had badly deteriorated over the four years too, although I'd done well with them. Many people with EB lose function way earlier than I did. Maybe it was luck, or perhaps the piano lessons I'd had as a kid had helped. I had always used my fingers constantly, even if they hurt. Regardless, eventually, the scarring took hold and my fingers began to fuse. My hands are usually wrapped in bandages now. I can still move the fingers a little – I can wiggle them and I can feel them. But I can't use them like I used to.

People see my hands and want to know, how do you write? How do you hold a cup? How do you hold your phone? Well, where there is a will there is a way! I believe it's about adapting. That's the key. No, I don't hold things in the way I used to; in fact, nothing in my life is the way it used to be. I could cry about it until the cows come home, but it wouldn't change anything. So I make do with what I can, and I look for workarounds – handles that work for me, stems on glasses, phone pops that I can put my thumb through. My biggest struggle will always be books, as I find it hard to turn the pages. But I still manage to do it. It's hard, but when you want something, you find a way to have it. I truly believe that.

Even as my hands are now – they've done so much. They've held the hands of little children. Typed out speeches. Sent texts. Reached for my mom's hand when we both needed steadying.

* * *

That year my parents booked to go to Los Angeles instead of our usual Florida, and we went to stay for a few weeks at the Hyatt hotel in Long Beach.

It was a whole new world.

The hotel was massive, and downstairs was open plan, with couches everywhere and a fancy bar I could roll right up to. I love LA for this – the inclusivity that's down to the fact that everywhere is so accessible. In Long Beach I was included everywhere, I could go into every building, I could go up every street. Nothing was a problem.

Back home in Ireland, beaches are out of bounds to wheelchair users. We can't get onto them at all; not even close in most places. But in LA I was made welcome.

Outside our hotel was a beautiful marina that we could walk to the beach along. It was called Long Beach and it lived up to its name. When we first got to the beach there I was overwhelmed. You see, I could go right onto the beach in my wheelchair. They had these long concrete pathways the length of the beach and right in the sand. They were designed for walking and bikes but also made for wheelchairs. It sounds small, but to me it meant everything.

Mom would stroll and I would roll in view of the water,

stopping for coffee, while Dad and Catherine would zoom off on bikes and cycle way ahead, and it felt really normal, more normal than I ever feel at home. It was a holiday for me in more ways than one.

LA is my favourite place on earth. I feel really calm there, because I can go anywhere and so I feel like I belong. For a while when I'm there, I get to live the life most people live, being able to just decide to go somewhere and go. That's what accessibility gives people: freedom. I don't feel like a burden in LA. I'm not stuck at a side door or searching and asking for ramps. Everything is already ready for me. It's like I matter. I'm included, I belong, and it hits me every time, because it's not like that in Europe, it's not like that in Ireland, where everything's a challenge.

I can't even go into my own bank in Portlaoise to use the account I've had since I was a teenager. I have to sit in the car while Mom goes in for me. *I'm* the customer. It's *my* money, but I can't access it on my own. Same for certain shops. I'll look in the window, see things I like and say to Mom or my PA, 'Can you go in and ask if that jumper comes in a size 10, size 12?'

I love clothes and I love shopping, but I can't always take part in the fun of it. If you are able-bodied, close your eyes and imagine my world for a moment – where you are physically prevented from entering places for no reason other than there is a physical barrier: steps. Shops, banks, friends' homes, venues, restaurants, bars. It's a game of pot luck, a world where often-times you won't realise you're shut out until you get there.

And so you can see why I love LA. We've been to loads of places, but if someone told me I'd a month to live I would book a flight there, straight away. LA will always be special to me.

***

Once, my family and I made the mistake of going to Barcelona. I really wanted to see it. Everybody I knew had been raving about it. A cultural hotspot and I wanted to go.

It *is* a gorgeous, gorgeous city, but my God, it is not for wheelchairs. Most streets are narrow and they can be cobbled. Even the Airbnb we were staying in was so awkward, with stairs to get in. And as for the metro, it is almost completely inaccessible. While you can get on at some stations, you cannot get off at others.

At one point, we were totally stuck underground, having got on the metro at an accessible station and off at another that wasn't. When we asked the station manager for help, he just shrugged and said, 'You will have to figure it out.' We were stuck at the bottom of this huge escalator with no way out of the station when a stranger saw us and stepped in. This Spanish man started wheeling me towards the escalator, then tilted my wheelchair to get me on. It was terrifying. I was shaking. Although grateful in a way, I was really, really angry that it had come to this.

I didn't see one other wheelchair user my whole time in Barcelona, not one. That says it all. It's not that there aren't people in Barcelona who need wheelchairs. They're there. But they're not out enjoying their own city. They're stuck inside, like I was for the rest of that trip.

You adapt in a wheelchair because you have to, but it's hard to be a grown-up when I have to rely on others for basic things, rely on my family, my PA or absolute strangers for help in and out of buildings that I *need* to get in and out of. I have no privacy. I can't go and blow all my money on ridiculously expensive boots and pretend they were on sale. Every single thing I do is witnessed, and it sucks. I can't sneak off to the cinema to watch some terrible movie on my own. I can't travel solo or have a quiet coffee by myself. I can pretend to, my PA would be happy to give me the experience and wait in the car, but she still has to drive me there. I can't run away. I can't do things without someone else involved. It's never an option.

If Ireland had real access, like they do in LA, I could live just like you. That's the bottom line.

People see my wheelchair, but I don't think they really see the truth of the limitations created by things that the able-bodied may recognise in that moment as tiny inconveniences without realising that these all stack up. People don't get it – unless you're in a wheelchair, you can't. You'll think it's just one step, just a curve, just a little thing. But it's not. It's the whole thing. It's the difference between being included in the world and being excluded. It's the difference between being independent and being at somebody's, everybody's, mercy.

So when I have to wait outside because of a step, I feel it. That's the part I'll never stop resenting. It's not that I hate being disabled. I just hate being really dependent on other people.

Accessibility isn't a favour. Accessibility isn't a kindness and it's not a special service.

It's a *right*, and it's *my* right.

And, yes, I'm still waiting for Ireland to catch up.

* * *

When I was ready and back on my feet, I started applying for jobs. My first interview was with the ESB. They didn't offer me the job, but it was a good experience. I didn't take it personally. The second interview was with Permanent TSB and I got the job, in the Head Office on Stephen's Green, Dublin, in the mortgage department.

Once that was sorted, I rented a room in the IFSC, living with five other girls in a huge apartment. Half of the roommates were rarely home, so I had a lot of space to myself. I liked it. It was quiet, down near the river. I had a lovely new PA who was from Dublin herself – Catherine – we got on *so* well. I love the way Dublin people gently slag you all the time. It makes you feel loved.

I made good friends with one of my roommates there, Sheila. When she was in we would grab dinner together in a place across the road that did chicken wings. She was so lovely. Other than those chicken wings, the only thing I could really eat at home was potato waffles – they were soft enough.

One time I came back and the waffle box was empty! 'Who ate my waffles?' I remember saying, and one of the roommates put her hand up.

'Sorry about that, Emma,' she said, 'I didn't know they were yours. I'll replace them.'

Well, I was raging. The only shop near us was an M&S Simply Food and there was nothing I could eat there!

Socially, I was still finding my feet. School had made me so reserved. And even though college helped somewhat, I was still figuring things out. I was still programmed by my teenage years to worry about what was coming and trying to predict what people were thinking.

In the mortgage centre the manager, Susan, showed me the

ropes. She explained how to take customer calls, how to look up files and use the systems. It was a lot.

'Do you want to try taking a call yourself now, Emma?' she said, after a couple of run-throughs.

'No!!' The word popped out of my mouth and surprised us both. But she was kind.

'Hmmm,' she said, 'let's sit you over here with this team, and you can take a call whenever you're feeling it.'

Over we went to a clump of desks at the back of the office. There were three guys there, each in a quarter of their own. She gave me the empty quarter of the circle and introduced me to the lads.

'Emma is going to shadow ye,' she told them. 'Emma, this is Ciaran, Shane and Evan. Oh and that's Adam.' She pointed to another guy at a desk a little bit away.

'Ciaran will show you the ropes,' Susan said.

'Grand,' Ciaran said and gave me a thumbs up.

That move was the best thing she could have done for me. Young lads in Ireland are always so easy-going, funny as hell, and these guys were really kind. Ciaran, who trained me in over the next few weeks, explained everything so clearly when he did it that it gave me the confidence to try myself. I could ask these lads questions without feeling stupid and, slowly, I started to feel a rhythm. I hadn't been around guys before. Girls' schools have a whole different energy and slagging was something that didn't really happen in our house! But these lads got me well used to how slagging worked pretty quickly.

'Fogarty's making the tea,' Adam would say, calling me by my last name all the time to make me laugh. I loved that. Being part of the laughter, instead of the reason for it, gave me great confidence.

The girls, who were in the next section, were lovely too: Sarah, Gwen and Catherine. They weren't on my team, but they'd stop by for chats a lot. I got really close with them.

In the bank, I never sat anyone down and explained EB to them. I wasn't ready and it didn't seem necessary. I think it was obvious that I had stuff I was dealing with. But they treated me like everyone else, and that was what I wanted.

I hadn't any experience in mixed groups, but the structure of the bank helped and gave me a way in. I was on a team, both in work and after it. There was a pub across the street from the bank, and most Friday evenings we'd all head over for drinks. I remember thinking, *So this is what independence feels like.* I was finally stepping into adult life – earning proper money, having weekend plans, building my own routine.

On that first Friday, I went home to change my clothes before meeting everyone, and by the time I got back out, I'd missed half the night. Lesson learned – change quickly with the other girls in work and go.

Once or twice I even ended up in Copper's. It's a Dublin institution, and a rite of passage for every Irish person. I'd always keep to the edges of the dance floor – always careful about physical contact – and the bank gang seemed to figure that out quickly. Without ever being instructed on EB care, they automatically and *always* made a ring around me. It was great. I could chat, dance, laugh along and not worry.

* * *

Head Office, where I worked, was not far from where Debra Ireland had just moved into a new office. I started dropping in there during my lunch breaks just to say hi to the girls I had got to know from the events we all would be at together. The first time I went, I walked the long way and ended up wrecked. Then I found a shortcut – a laneway just outside the office that led right to Debra's door. It took me five minutes and I couldn't believe my luck!

After that, a visit to Debra became part of my day. I'd go in for a chat or to lend a hand. Clyde was there, of course, but there was also a gang of girls my age working: Kim, Caitriona and Lynn. They already, of course, knew all about EB and it was a huge part of their lives. I watched the clock for lunchtime, so I could get over to help out there and catch up with them. I never had to explain, never had to pretend. We became really close friends.

After work I'd maybe do a quick bit of shopping, then I would get the bus (or sometimes a taxi) back to my apartment on the quays. It doesn't sound like much, but it meant everything to me. I was part of the world, not just someone watching out a window.

A year and a half later, I moved to Inchicore, to this little two-bed that the landlord had for his daughters. One room was mine, one was theirs, but they were rarely, if ever, there.

I got a new PA, Jackie. She would make me coddle because I could eat it. I loved her, she was great at bandages. I was really living the good life: working, friends, places to be. I was travelling, speaking, choosing my clothes, saying what I wanted to say. I was figuring out who I was.

But ...

I started to realise I wouldn't outpace EB. I *couldn't*. No matter how busy or upbeat I was, EB was the boss of me. EB held all the cards. EB would always catch up with me.

You see, as a child and later as a teenager, I never thought

EB could stop me from living the life I pictured. I thought I'd go to college, then I'd fall in love, then I'd get married and have kids. That's what people did. That was life, right?

I believed it just like everyone else.

I stayed in that mindset for a long time, and, honestly, I'm glad I did, because I got to have the same moments everyone else had – the butterflies when someone I liked walked by, the laughs with friends, the daydreams. I felt like a normal girl.

I still do, in some ways.

That mindset didn't really shift until I was in my mid-twenties.

I began to think about what being married would actually look like for me. What would it mean for someone else to live with EB too? All my care. The dressings. The pain. The stress. And I thought, *How could I ever ask someone to take that on?*

It isn't that I don't think I'm worth loving. I am. I know I am. I just know how much it would take out of someone to be with me and that just never sat right.

Once I saw that clearly, I couldn't pretend I hadn't.

There's a lot of joy in love. A lot of hope. But EB complicates everything. It isn't just hard, it takes over and affects everything. I didn't want EB to take over someone else's life the way it has mine.

So I let that dream go, a little at a time. Not all at once. That might have killed me.

I had told myself that if I kept moving, I could stay ahead of the hard parts, but it doesn't work like that. Sometimes I still think about those early dreams. Daddy walking me down the aisle. A bunch of kids in my back seat instead of a wheelchair. Travelling the world. Dancing in the rain with my sister.

Those dreams are still living inside me, they still look for my attention sometimes when I am drifting away in my imagination into that land where I don't have EB and I am just Emma. I cry for the loss of them, for what EB has stolen from me.

I know those dreams are lost.

But I've made new ones too.

Dreams where I speak and am heard. Dreams where something I say or do makes a difference. Where I change minds. Where someone with EB sees me and knows they're not alone. That life won't be easy, but it will still be *theirs*.

I've lost things.

But I've kept more than I thought I would.

I've lost things, but I have found amazing treasures. That matters more than anything else.

And I was starting to understand that.

18

Butterfly

Not all turning points are dramatic.

Mine definitely wasn't.

I had stopped in to see my aunt and I was walking up the slope to her door when I heard a sharp crack. I wasn't sure what it was, thinking it could have been my shoe hitting against a stone. I definitely did consider that it might be my foot. I'd broken it like that before, but I didn't feel any pain, so I just carried on.

To be honest I forgot about it and the next day when my foot was sore and aching I just thought it was the usual aches of EB. That's what I keep coming back to. People think something big must have happened for me to go from my own two feet to a wheelchair. But it was just a misstep, a wrong angle, the kind of thing *you* shrug off a hundred times in your life.

That weekend, at home in Mom and Dad's, I couldn't walk at all. On the Monday I rang in sick and went to the hospital. It took an MRI to see that the damage, the cause of the pain, was a hairline crack that ran the length of one of the bones in my foot. I remember thinking, *Okay, that sounds like nothing*. But it wasn't nothing.

An EB specialist confirmed it. 'This is the worst kind of fracture for someone in your situation,' he said.

Even with that, I was hopeful. I told myself I'd be back at work soon. And for a while, I really believed that. I really, really believed it.

A blister opened on the same foot and got infected. The bone refused to heal. It became this game of wait, recover, try again. Permanent TSB held my place for a while because I kept saying I'd be back. I kept on the flat in Dublin too, even though the rent was high, for as long as I could, but I couldn't keep it up. I had something else to worry about too – the knowledge that I'd lose my current PA if I moved outside the Dublin boundary.

I would make progress, then go backwards. I'd start improving, then be back to square one. Everything I built for myself, the job, the independence – it was all gone.

One step. That's all it took. I went from working full-time, living independently, to lying in bed back in my parents' house.

I kept repeating the same line over and over again: 'I can't believe this happened.'

I kept waiting for someone to say, 'Emma, stop overreacting, you will be absolutely fine again soon.'

But they never did.

I never went back to the bank. Technically, I could have worked from a wheelchair. But I relied on buses and taxis, and even that wasn't easy.

Eventually I gave in. I moved home. I said a tearful goodbye to Jackie and I met a new PA, Eileen. She was wonderful and we had a fantastic relationship, but it was hard.

My world changed again. I lost touch with people. That happens.

Over time, my wheelchair has become part of my life, but I'll be honest with you, I really hate it. I have never got used to it.

I do have one with a motor, but those chairs are impossible to put into a car and I want to go out, so I have to be pushed.

I hate being so low down when everyone's standing and I'm sitting. The conversation floats above my head and I can't hear half of it. I'm left out. It's not on purpose, it's not intentional, but it still happens, and it does hurt. I hate when I'm wheeled up to a high table of a bar with people sitting around on stools, and the only thing I can see are people's belt buckles and elbows. You don't feel part of what's going on; you feel like a child. And there's no slipping into a room quietly when you're being pushed, when you're in a wheelchair – you enter and everybody notices. The room parts like the Red Sea when I come through it and I find it really embarrassing.

And the thing is, that chair, that difference, it isolates you even in the most simple human moments, such as when my uncle passed away. Mom came flying into my room. 'Your uncle passed away, Emma,' she said, and then she ran straight back out. I just lay there alone with the news and no way to run after her.

Another time I heard Mom shouting and there some kind of commotion. Daddy had fallen in the river near our house and very nearly drowned, coming home soaked and scared. I could hear my very upset father, and my mother sounded hysterical, but I couldn't even go out into the hall and I had no idea what the matter was. I just had to wait.

In those moments I am outside of life. I am listening through a wall, present, but not part of it. It's nobody's fault, but I feel useless. I feel *useless*, and I hate saying this, because I know I'm not, but that's how I *feel* a lot of the time. Like I'm surplus, like the story is happening without me.

It's nobody's fault when my mom puts my dad first because

he needs her to. But if I could walk, I could have been there for my dad too.

***

People will say to me, 'Oh, I've a terrible headache,' and then immediately go, 'Sorry, I shouldn't complain in front of you.' Listen, you're allowed to be in pain. Just because I'm already in pain doesn't mean your pain isn't valid. We all experience it.

My dad will say things like, 'She's used to it,' and I'm like, 'No!'

Have I got used to pain? That's something I don't know how to answer, but I don't think so. I don't think my brain cares or even knows that I've felt this way since birth. It fires signals just like anyone. Pain is pain. I suffer and I look for relief.

Before my twenties, though, I could get by with paracetamol, maybe a bit of ibuprofen if things were bad. If I had a really bad wound, I could take both. I knew my body back then. It felt like I had a sort of agreement with it: you hurt, but I'll manage.

Then came my mid-twenties and it was like a switch flicked. I'd always had wounds, always needed care, but my body – well, it had some sort of grit to it before then. Some natural endurance of youth that faded around twenty-five. Suddenly the pain began to stack up.

Things became unbearable.

Bobby and I compared notes all the time – on pain, on meds, on new tricks and techniques. The way I saw it was that Bobby was three years ahead of me, so he knew every step of this that other people could only imagine. Nobody got it like Bobby.

I think as well, subconsciously, that is why I loved to see how independent and future-focused Bobby was. He was building his own house, he had a girlfriend, he was always travelling and doing things. Bobby's pain had advanced like mine was starting to.

On his advice, I started seeing a pain specialist. It was a hard moment, walking into a room and admitting, finally, 'This is too much.' I had to accept that the pain was changing me. And it wasn't going away.

I remember one of my first prescriptions made me so relaxed I could have floated away. And it made me chatty. I'd talk for hours non-stop, drowsy, in the sitting room with everyone, just nattering away. I don't remember most of it, but Mom and Catherine do. They nicknamed it 'Emma's Talky Talk Time'. Catherine says she would be trying to watch *Coronation Street* or whatever, and I'd start up from the corner of the room, cosily delivering my whole life story.

'Oh God,' she'd mutter, 'here she goes.'

Herself and Mom would turn up the telly and throw me the odd 'uh huh' or 'I see.'

They never minded, of course they didn't, not even when I talked through the ads and well into the next show before I finally succumbed to sleep. Kim says I once spoke non-stop for three hours.

'You were off on your own planet,' she laughs.

Those early meds, they gave me some peace in a heavy time. But that was then. Now, at forty-one, I've tried nearly everything. Morphine patches, tramadol, codeine, nerve blockers. I've maxed out the doses I'm allowed. There's no 'up' left to go. I tried a pain-relief lollipop once, but it not only tasted awful, it tore the inside of my cheek to bits. So that was that.

Most days, pain relief medication barely scratches the surface. Some days it's not bearable. Some days I am barely able to speak. It gets so bad that I can't even look at my phone. I just lie with my eyes shut and try to bear it. My pain is layered now, and it's unpredictable. It burns, it stabs, it's white heat. It can feel like glass. Sometimes I feel like I am being dipped in boiling water. Other times, it's like someone's taken a knife to me and is twisting it, slowly.

Doctors say that living with EB is like living with third-degree burns that never heal. And they're right.

There's no real rest.

But on top of that, I have to change my bandages daily, no matter what. People with EB are susceptible to skin cancer and sepsis, so those two things are always watched for during bandage changes. And I often have to go through procedures. If something isn't right, it gets looked into – and unfortunately for me that means more pain.

When I was twenty-five I had had this rough lump on my foot for ages. It was around the size of a 50p piece and my dermatologist wasn't happy with it, but I wasn't too worried. This was just another of my long-standing battles with my feet.

'Emma, I need to take a better look,' the dermatologist said, just after Christmas. I knew what that meant. A biopsy. I hated those.

Bobby commiserated when I told him.

'Me too,' he said, 'I just had one on my hand.' He'd been there, done that before me every time.

'It's never-ending,' I said.

Biopsies always had to be done because skin cancer and EB go hand in hand. Our skin is wounded so often and heals so poorly, it becomes fertile ground for mutations. Bobby had explained that to me once – he knew so much about it because he had already had skin cancer six times.

'Our skin regenerates so quickly,' he told me, 'that's how it starts.'

There was nothing I was going through that he hadn't. Well, except for heartbreak, which he was also dealing with at that time, freshly dumped by his girlfriend. He was more cut up about that than anything else. Those were the real-life moments. Not EB.

EB always felt run-of-the-mill, even when it was being difficult.

'So what have they said?' he asked.

I told him they had frozen it, scraped it and put acid on it. Nothing had made a difference.

'They want to do a biopsy of course,' I said, 'as per usual, but I'm not sure. They always do them, and it's always nothing.'

'Come on, Emma,' he said, 'just get it done and it will be done.'

He was right. So I went to the hospital, lay on the table and let them give me six anaesthetic injections to the sides of my heel as they tried to numb it and give me pain relief at the same time. They may as well have given me nothing. Mom said she could hear me screaming down the corridor. She said she nearly stormed in to stop them. But they did it, regardless, and took the patch off. And people wonder why I hate the hospital.

'When are your results back?' I asked Bobby one night about a week later.

'Next week,' he said. 'Yours?'

'I'm hoping to hear today,' I said. 'I really hope they won't want to do any more this year.'

Later I got a call. All clear. I'd suspected all was well, but I was still relieved. And, of course, I texted Bobby straight away.

'Brilliant,' he said and we changed the subject. Back to the main topic of most people our age: love.

'I had a lovely present for her and everything,' he said of his ex.

So I did the usual, offered advice, listened, let him rant.

'The house is finished,' he said, 'Pool table in situ in the living room ... And she dumps me.'

I tried to think of the perfect thing to say – he was so miserable.

'She's missing out,' I consoled him. 'I can't wait to see the house anyway. I can't believe you did it! You've moved out. You always wanted to!'

He cheered up a bit.

'All we need is to get you driving now, Emma,' he scolded.

'I tried!' I told him.

I *had* tried.

I had gone for a couple of driving lessons with the Irish Wheelchair Association years earlier, when I was around twenty-two, but the car wasn't adapted for someone like me in any way, and I just couldn't put my trust in it. The instructor was so lovely and patient, but she was constantly grabbing the wheel.

'This isn't driving!' I'd say to her, half-laughing, half-panicking. She'd laugh too, but I think we both knew the truth – we were trying to fit a square peg into a round hole. It just wasn't working. One of us had to admit it. So I stopped going.

'I know,' Bobby said, 'but you gave up! Don't give up.'

He always had my back, even when I didn't agree. This time was no different.

'Emma, you have to get back out there,' Bobby said. '*Carpe diem*.'

A week later there were a few days where I didn't hear from Bobby. My texts to him sat unread. I wondered about it and figured he might be busy, or maybe his phone wasn't working or his internet was down. I pushed a nagging thought away. His new house would be taking up his time. Maybe he was working things out with the girlfriend.

I'll hear from him soon.

And I did.

But when contact restored, it was a call flashing up instead of a message.

My heart stopped. Bobby never rang. We were texters. Always had been.

Something was wrong.

19

Forever Young

'Hey.'

Bobby's voice was calm. So I didn't panic straight away. We talked about something random. Then there was a pause.

'My results came back,' he said.

I went cold. You know that feeling, when your stomach drops? I felt it.

'It's cancer,' he said. I held my breath. Bobby had had cancer before. It would be okay.

'What kind?' I said.

'Squamous cell carcinoma,' he told me and the world tilted. That was the aggressive form. A gasp came from me.

'I've a year,' he said, 'maybe a bit more if I'm lucky.'

I cried out loud down the phone. I couldn't help it.

He said he needed to call a few other people, so I let him go and sat there in silence, tears rolling down my face. Mom came in, saw my face and knelt down on the floor beside me.

'What happened?' she asked.

I told her. We stayed there for ages, just repeating ourselves.

'This can't be happening.'

'Not Bobby.'

I felt shattered in a way that had nothing to do with my

body. I couldn't imagine life without Bobby's messages, his jokes, his sideways take on everything; I didn't want it.

Bobby had always been there. Always.

Even when I was a baby, he was ahead of me on the path proving there was life in this disease. Bobby was the reason my parents had hope.

And now he was *leaving*? Like this?

The injustice of it sat on my chest like a weight. Why him? Why not someone else? Why someone so bright and kind and bloody brilliant? I wanted to scream into the sky.

* * *

Bobby kept me updated as the months went by, little by little. I went down to Limerick whenever I could, and I saw the beautiful house that he had built. It was the kind of place you imagine a person building when they want peace, space and sky. That house was a life's goal ticked off. I was so proud of him.

He handled his illness with this quiet grace, the same way he handled EB. No drama. No fuss. With truth and his motto flying fierce: seize the day.

Debra Ireland booked him a surprise – a Ferrari rental – so he could live another dream, to drive a real sports car. Bobby loved his cars. He had a ball. He booked himself two holidays, one with his parents and one with his PA on a cruise. The stories from that trip made me laugh so much. We made plans for good things; we thought he had time. We found out that Michael Jackson, his musical hero, was coming to Dublin and I sat up waiting for the ticket lines to open to make sure he got to go.

Bobby was my best friend, planning things was normal, but

it felt so surreal to be planning fun times with him which had this looming edge to them. These times would be the last times. That early part of 2009 was one of the darkest times of my life. I can't imagine what Bobby felt because he never showed it. But for me there was a ticking clock on my best friend's life – it felt terrifying. I would wake up each morning knowing I was one day closer to losing someone who understood me in a way nobody else ever had.

Bobby organised a casino night at his house, so we could all dress up in black tie and have fun together. There were gambling tables and cocktails, he knew exactly what he wanted from it. He had a digital frame set up, with photos of all of us scrolling past as we chatted and laughed. It was beautiful. Even though he was really feeling his illness by that stage, he still played the perfect host and made sure everyone had the best time, his house full of colour and chaos and laughter. He even made a speech.

'One cure for a broken heart anyway,' he said during it, 'is to be told you've cancer.' It made us all smile, even though none of this was funny. Even in the darkest times Bobby tried to keep it light.

I met a little EB baby, Liam, the day after the party. His mom, Grainne, had brought him down for it. He wasn't even one and those big baby eyes made my heart melt. And those lashes! I still remember thinking, *He's the most beautiful little boy I've ever seen*. For all the pain and heartache he was already going through, he was so calm, so content. I just had to have a cuddle. I knew how fragile he was – his skin like mine – but he was too cute not to hold. I was gentle, and he just sat there on my lap, completely at peace, looking up at me with those big eyes. I melted.

Bobby leaned in to say hello to Liam and welcome him to the family. As he did, someone snapped a photo and we laughed our heads off when we saw it.

'Look at this,' he said, sending it to me later, 'everyone is calling us the EB family.'

That made me laugh so much. I shared it with everyone. After that, we became the EB family.

It's the little things like that isn't it?

A message from a friend.

A house party with people who love you.

A laugh with a pal.

***

That was May. We started planning for my birthday in June.

About a week later, I remember, I went down to see Bobby. My PA Eileen went too, and when we arrived Bobby came outside and said, 'Come run errands with me, I've to collect something.'

That was nothing new. He had this sporty car and we would often drive around singing along to Michael Jackson's greatest hits playing on the radio.

Next thing I knew we were pulling into this massive empty lot beside some warehouse near the college. He stopped the car in the middle of it and turned to me.

'Right,' he said, 'your turn.'

I knew what he meant, but I still said, 'What?'

'You're going to drive, Emma.'

There was no way I was going to take him up on this. It was way too scary a prospect.

'What's my motto?' he said.

I stared at him. I knew what it was. He always said it whenever something was up for debate.

'Emma,' he said, 'what is my motto?'

'*Carpe diem*,' I said, my voice shaking.

He smiled and got out of the car.

Seize the day.

Somehow, heart hammering in my chest, I swapped seats and took the wheel. I drove like a disaster, round in a circle. It was jerky and messy, but I did it. And I knew, in that moment, I wanted to drive.

That was Bobby. That was what he gave me.

* * *

The last time I saw Bobby was at his home, set high on a hill, the beautiful Limerick countryside all around. Of course, I didn't know it would be the last time.

When I pulled up outside and saw him come to the door, my heart stopped. He looked *wrecked*. Not the worn-out I'd seen before, tired from work or stressed-out from exams. He was worn through, as if something inside him had already started switching off and there was no stopping it. Tears pricked the back of my eyes so I looked away, out the window at the view instead of at him. I stared at the trees and the hedges and I cried without him seeing.

The emotion I felt was hard to describe. Because yes, Bobby was my best friend – without a doubt, one of the closest people in my life – but at the same time, every time I looked at him, especially near the end, I felt like I was looking at my own future. That's the truth of it. That was the scariest part. Watching someone you love disappear in slow motion and knowing somewhere deep in your gut, *this could be me*. This *will* be me, maybe. Not now, not next year – but someday. That kind of thought doesn't just sit with you. It presses on your chest.

We sat, Mom and I, with Bobby and his family, and we had tea. I watched him fading from the moment we arrived. Mom and I looked at each other, knowing we should probably go and let him rest, but when we stood up to say so, Bobby totally panicked, like a child being left alone would. He begged us to stay.

'Please,' he said, something almost breaking in his voice. 'It's just the medication making me drowsy. I'll be grand. Please, please, Emma, Pat, just don't go yet.'

We gladly sat back down. Of course we did. We had lunch with his mom and sister, a lovely lasagne.

Even as he nodded off, we stayed and talked a bit more, but the day drew on and, finally, I hugged Bobby goodbye.

I didn't know it would be the last time I'd see him. He had been given a year in February and it was only mid-June. We had plans for my birthday, meeting up in town, dolled up, with all my friends. He fully intended to be there.

But maybe a part of me did know, somewhere deep in my heart, because when we hugged goodbye I found it really hard to let go.

Bobby passed away a few days later, on my birthday.

Nothing can ever take that pain away. Not even the strongest medication in the world.

* * *

On the morning of my birthday a howl burst out of me as I woke. I hadn't even opened my eyes properly, but I knew.

I *knew*.

Mom was on the phone downstairs. In my sleep I'd heard her say, 'Will you come home?' So I knew. I started to cry before I'd even fully woken up.

I heard Mom say, quietly, 'I have to go, I think Emma knows.'

Bobby was gone. My best friend. My confidant. My partner in this mad world of EB. I'd never get a message from him again. I'd never see his name flash up on my phone. I'd never catch his eye at a Debra event when someone's speech was going on too long or they were saying something mad. I'd never hear his voice. I'd never laugh again the way I did with him.

Grief isn't just in your mind or in your heart, it's all over. It sits in your throat and behind your eyes and in your chest all at once. It's in your hands.

I cried all day. Mom sat beside me and just held my hand and rubbed my head like she used to, when I was a baby in pain.

Then the phone rang again. My aunty Angela this time.

'Did you hear who else passed away today?' she said.

Mom said, 'What? Who?' She was so confused.

'Just turn on *Sky News*,' my aunt said.

Mom turned on the telly and there it was. Michael Jackson had also passed away that day.

We just kept saying the same words to each other: 'This can't be real.'

You know, there was something strange and comforting about that. Bobby and I had tickets to see him. We were meant to go together. Now the concert wasn't happening and that felt right to me. And now they were eternally linked, those two names – Michael Jackson and his biggest fan, Bobby.

Both gone. Both legends in their own way.

I didn't have to call to cancel the things we had booked for my birthday. Kim rang and neither of us even considered going ahead with anything. Clyde rang too, and when he said happy birthday it felt like there was no such thing as birthdays at all. Then Mom said, 'Emma, I have your presents.' It seemed so bizarre to open presents, but I was really moved to see that she had bought me a digital frame, just like the one Bobby had.

* * *

Bobby's funeral was at his house. They laid him out on his beloved pool table, in the same room we'd sat in together only a few weeks back. When I walked in and saw the people I knew, the gang we used to see at Debra events, there was a second where it felt normal. Like maybe Bobby would be out in a minute with a cheeky grin.

But then I saw the coffin. He wasn't going to arrive.

Bobby was dead.

This was a room Bobby designed – it had the pool table, a little bar he'd nicknamed 'Bob's Bar', a jukebox and all those bits and pieces he'd collected over the years. *He* was in that room. His *life* was in that room. The joy of it, the memories, the laughs.

Maybe it should have felt comforting, but it felt like a terrible joke.

The house was full, people everywhere, but it felt so empty.

Katherine Sweeney, a nurse who had cared for us in St James's Hospital, came over to me and wrapped her arms around me. 'I'm so proud of you,' she said. 'I'm so proud of you, Emma.'

I couldn't even speak. I wanted to say something, anything,

but I felt like I wasn't in my body, like I was outside of myself, watching it all unfold from somewhere far away. It was like a dream that was so vivid it felt real but too surreal to bear.

I kept thinking, *Am I really here? Is this happening? Is Bobby really gone?*

I was in Bobby's house, standing beside Bobby's pool table, looking at all the things he loved. His car was outside, his front door was open. This was his dream. But Bobby was gone. And I didn't know what to do with that. I still don't.

I went to his parents and his sister Suzi, who is a nurse in Dublin. I hugged them. I held them. I told them I was sorry. These are the things we do. I spoke softly. I didn't mention his name.

All of the other people there were doing the same. I could see it in their eyes, the way they blinked, the way their hands wouldn't stay still. All trying to be strong. Me trying to be strong. And in the middle of all that trying, we just came together, all broken bits and grief and love, clinging to each other like people trying not to drown.

My words came out scrambled, but so did theirs. I was crying and smiling at the same time, saying things I don't even remember. So were they. But that's grief, isn't it? It scrambles the signal.

I saw so many mutual friends in the room that day. There were others too. His friends from home: Niall, Marie, Sandra. His cousins Sandra and Karen. They all felt the loss so deeply – you could see the profound grief on their faces.

We could barely look at each other. It's said all the time, but death is *so* final. And the death of a young person is unfair. None of us needed to say that out loud to make it true. We were all holding a piece of Bobby, but the truth was we had nothing.

Maybe that's how we carry on. By holding those pieces we are left with forever.

Just before they took Bobby to the church, I went over and looked at him. He was dressed in a suit, with an old pocket watch in the top pocket. I kissed my hand and placed it on his chest. But I couldn't speak any words, there was nothing in any language that could express my sorrow.

At the church, they placed Bobby's coffin off to the side, which struck me. Maybe that was his wish, maybe it's the way it's done in that parish, I don't know. But it made it harder.

On the back of the Mass pamphlet, they had printed his motto: *Seize the Day*.

At the grave, they lowered the coffin down into the earth and I burst into tears. And then came the part I will never forget. In that part of Ireland your people will join together to bury you. I was used to walking away before the gravediggers came. But here, the family, friends and neighbours began the job themselves. One by one, thunk thunk thunk, they threw soil onto the lid of his coffin. And each stone that hit the wood felt like a bullet straight into my heart.

I wanted to shout. I wanted to beg them, 'Stop it! Don't you know how soft he is? How gentle he was?'

But I didn't. I stood still, the noise in my ears louder than any I'd ever heard.

Bobby had told me the cure for heartbreak was to get cancer. I learned that was true.

Two weeks later, I was diagnosed with cancer myself.

20

The Moment I Knew

About ten days after they removed it, the lump on my foot had come back and the doctors were flummoxed.

'We need to remove the entire area,' they said.

My mother stood up and her arms flew out across me.

'You will be giving her a general anaesthetic,' she said, 'you're not doing it under local.'

They agreed. I don't think any of us wanted to go through that again.

'Are you worried?' I said, trying to read the dermatologist's face.

He didn't seem to be. 'Not really,' he said, 'but I want to look at this thing properly. It has me baffled.'

Just after Bobby's funeral, we were called into the hospital for results and a chat. I would normally be really nervous getting a call like that, but I think grief had stripped me of any feeling. I felt as calm as anything when I was checked in.

Then the doctor came in, glanced at me and turned to the others. 'Could you give me a moment with Emma?'

'I'm staying,' Mom said.

'Emma,' the doctor said, 'you have skin cancer.'

A thought came into my head: *Of course. Of course this is happening.*

A nurse brought me in a cup of tea straight away. That's what we do, isn't it? Tea is the old Irish fix for everything.

I didn't react how even I would have expected. I'd already spent all my tears on Bobby. When I heard the words, I just went numb, because I had just watched cancer dismantle the friend I cherished most in the world.

But that also gave me something to hold on to. I kept telling myself, *this is only the beginning.* If Bobby had faced it seven times, then I could face it this first time. I imagined myself at a theme park, roller coaster ahead of me, just starting the ride. It helped, in a strange way. Bobby's story became my grip on the lap bar, the thing that steadied me.

'The best cure for heartbreak is to get cancer,' he'd said, and we'd all laughed with him, because it was dark and ridiculous and awful.

But he'd meant it as well, in such a sad way. Bobby's life was so much more valuable than any relationship: he wanted to live. Now here I was, just a few weeks after he'd passed away, sitting in a hospital with a cup of warm tea in my hands, wondering if maybe he'd been right.

It *was* true, because once the diagnosis came, the grief was pushed aside. We don't have enough space in our heads for both. Instead of mourning Bobby, I clung to his life.

'I'll get to twenty-eight,' I said out loud like a manifesto. I was twenty-five. I had cancer and Bobby was gone. Bobby had been twenty-eight.

I would follow his path like I always had and make it to twenty-eight.

The rest of what cancer brought – paperwork, scans, blood tests – that all blurred into one long string of nods and reassurances that never quite got in.

'This is really treatable,' the doctor told me, 'it was an early catch.'

I would be okay.

And I was. A week later I went to Bobby's month's mind.

I got through that first bout of cancer with a kind of focus I didn't know I had. There was determination in me, and a deep refusal to let it win. There was also a lot of anger. I was so furious that having EB wasn't enough, that now I had this as well. The universe surely had made a mistake. Surely I was only ever supposed to have one burden? But life doesn't play fair. Not for me anyway.

Bobby still finds his way back to me. Not like Nana did, not as a smiling face in the light at night-time, but in the ordinary details of life – when I see a car like his, or when I hear Michael Jackson. The smell of a certain cologne. Photos, memories popping up unexpectedly on my phone. He comes through to me with the continued friendship I have with his family, in his sister Suzi popping her head around the door in the hospital where she is a nurse and I am often a patient. Suzi lived with EB her whole early life through Bobby, and she went into nursing because of him.

Sometimes, when I'm feeling really scared to put myself out there or do something I don't think I can do, I can hear his voice in my mind telling me to go on: *Go on, Emma, carpe diem, seize the day.*

* * *

I'd lost my best friend, I'd lost my independence and I was dealing with a new life in a wheelchair. It seemed like everything was changing.

Debra Ireland was also going through a change. They had a new CEO, Jimmy Fearon, who had come on board with them in the months just before Bobby passed away. God love him starting out with all that grief, totally misunderstanding the quiet in the office for a lack of drive, as he bounced in full of ideas, enthusiastic as can be. Deirdre had to pull him aside and explain that he would have to wait a while before kicking off his new campaigns.

Towards the end of the year, my mom suggested I go up to Dublin one or two days a week to volunteer there.

'I think it will do you the world of good,' she said, 'you know all the girls and you can help.'

'They probably don't need anyone,' I said.

'Don't be silly,' Mom said, 'charities always need volunteers.'

'I'd only get in the way,' I said.

I think I was still making excuses when my mom pushed my wheelchair onto the train and waved me off.

One of the girls from Debra, I think it was Kim, collected me that first morning. And that became the routine. I'd go up and spend the day answering phones and doing small admin jobs, and that work, plus the company of the girls, was like actual medicine.

That idea that my mom had, little did we know, was the beginning of so much.

I'd always say hello to Jimmy when he passed, but I didn't get to know him until one night we sat beside each other at a Debra event. We started chatting and didn't stop. He had great ideas. So did I.

The next week he came down to my desk, where I was answering phones.

'I've an idea, Emma,' Jimmy said, 'would you consider answering donations with a personal thank you?'

'I'd love to!' I said.

His idea was that I would write to donors and express how much it meant to get their support. That came easy to me, because I meant each and every one – and I always made it personal, because, for me, it really is personal. Their money helps people like me with EB now, and their money and time and effort helps move the world towards a time where EB won't exist.

The feedback to Jimmy was amazing.

'We need to put our heads together more,' Jimmy said. Then he said, 'Would you be up for just doing what you're already doing but on a more formal level?'

When he said that my heart soared. I realised what was happening. I was finding a path among all of this pain. I had a reason. Patient Ambassador. I would give this my all.

'I just mean you'd keep writing emails,' he said when I didn't answer. 'You know, keep attending events, sharing your story but formally, as a Patient Ambassador?'

He took my lack of response as reluctance. 'We can pay your travel expenses!' he added in a rush.

But he wouldn't have had to. As I got my breath back, I said a firm yes.

It felt like a job, but not in the way I'd had in the bank, where the names on the screen were meaningless. Here, these names, they were people like me, or people who wanted to help us. I have so many friends from Debra Ireland. Aoife and Sarah, for example, they're supporters rather than staff. They do a lot of fundraising and stay involved in that way. Then there's my lovely friend Jude – she worked there too, as head of fundraising.

Most of the friends I have now, I've met because of work, or the charity, or EB in some way. That's how it goes. I was close to the girls in the office, but it wasn't just about friendship – it was about the work. There was a sense of purpose, a kind of shared commitment. A door to who I was meant to be.

My wheelchair had felt like such an end point, but here I was in a new beginning.

One day, months later, Jimmy decided to look through old emails, lists and donations to check that we hadn't missed an opportunity. We had. We had missed a connection with the actor Colin Farrell.

Jimmy and I gawped at each other.

'Did nobody follow up on that?' he said in disbelief. It was disappointing to realise nobody had.

'Okay, so nobody did back then,' I said. 'Let's just contact him now.'

Jimmy reached out and hoped for a reply.

And, incredibly, Colin replied straight away – he wanted to do something with us. We were absolutely delighted.

People like Colin can do a lot for a charity. We knew it, and we knew Colin knew it. So, of course, we wanted to say thank you.

Thank you so much, I wrote back, and I acknowledged that his support would encourage more of it from others. This was an incredible opportunity for the charity.

At the time we were getting numbers together for a mini marathon, and the team came up with a great idea: the five women who raised the most money would all have dinner together with a special guest: Colin Farrell.

The project was launched, then and there, on radio and daytime shows, and I think every woman in Ireland started campaigning, but sure, look, would you blame them? Colin is an icon.

I could not wait to meet him.

21

Daylight

For people who know me, it's easy. I don't feel like a burden. But for people who don't know me, I think there's still that hesitation, a kind of nervousness about how to help.

That soon fades, thank God, and before I know it, usually, people get into the swing of it. I love making new friends, but I'm always glad when they figure me out. I'm tougher than they think.

In saying that, in the Debra office I had friends who not only liked me but understood *everything* about EB without me having to explain it. All of a sudden I had a life full of people who included me and wanted me around.

I had purpose. I had a path. I had a reason to get up in the mornings. Everything I had suffered and gone through had led me here. To this point.

It also brought me something else I had always wanted. Female community.

Kim, Caitriona, Lynn and I would go out, stay in each other's houses and generally just be girls together. I got to know their families, their other friends.

After nights out, Lynn would often drive me home. It's a forty-five minute drive from Dublin, but she would do record times because she drives like a maniac! She would blast the music and we would sing along, to *Glee*, to Adele, anything we could find.

Some Sunday mornings I'd find myself waking up on one of the girls' couches, and I'd be handed a cup of tea by one of their parents, or we would wake up in the same room and laugh until we were sick at stories of how funny we'd been the night before.

Just like every other girl my age.

We used to travel across to Wicklow for a Debra event that was on every year called the Wicklow Challenge. It was an event that brought supporters, athletes, patients and their families together – those events are my favourite (though I love a fancy night out just as much), always fun and meaningful. The Wicklow Challenge was an endurance hike up into the Wicklow Mountains, along a route set by Ronan, our guide. Ronan is a real character – part mountain-man, part athlete – who knows the mountains like the back of his hand. It wasn't easy, but it had a kind of reverence about it. Athletes would take it on as a test of endurance and fitness. Ray D'Arcy did a lot for us with that challenge, he was great to us.

Since Covid it hasn't happened, and I really miss it. I'd stay overnight at Lynn's house. I'd sleep on the couch in the kitchen, and I loved it. It felt safe and familiar. Her family were so welcoming – people would be coming in and out, saying hello, and I felt completely at ease.

We do the Kerry Challenge now – three days of hiking through the Dingle Peninsula – and we always make a weekend of it, which, of course, brings us all to the pub in the evening. That usually involves a lot of singing.

There was one night during the Kerry Challenge when Lynn wasn't there but her parents were. We'd been in the pub, and I was heading back to the hotel with Caitriona and Kim. As we were leaving, there was a step outside. Lynn's dad offered to help me. Well, he started off gentle – so careful and sweet – and then suddenly he took off, belting down a ramp and up the road with me in the wheelchair. I could hear him chuckling away and I thought, *If there's one tiny bump ahead, I'm on my face.* Kim and Caitriona were screaming, half laughing, half begging him to stop. I was laughing too, but I didn't know if it was from joy or sheer terror.

It's that pure Irish madness. You're laughing, thinking, *We absolutely should not be doing this* – but you do it anyway. There's something in that chaos that just lifts your soul.

Craic – that sort of laughter and lightness – you can't buy it. In Ireland, thank God, we have it in spades.

There was another time when I went out with the girls, and, for whatever reason, I ended up staying alone in a hotel for the first time, which, when you can't walk, sounds absolutely mental now that I write it down. The girls brought me back to the hotel that night and, with a few drinks on board, formed a team to help me take my medication and get me ready for bed. The three of them tucked me in, and we could not stop laughing and messing.

One of the girls – I won't say who – got the giggles when she was helping to give me my pain medication. When she lifted the syringe up, some of the medication dribbled along the heel of her hand and she licked it without thinking.

'Oh my God!' I tried to sound stern, but I had the giggles too. 'What are you doing?'

She looked at me, deadpan. 'What was in that?'

I nearly fell out of the bed laughing, but I wouldn't tell her what it was.

The girls ended up chatting to me for so long that they missed the last bus by two hours and had to get a taxi. The next morning one of them came, got me dressed and brought me to the train.

The medication licker rang me just before the train got into Portlaoise and said, 'Emma, what did I lick off my hand last night?'

And I said, 'Do you *really* want to know?'

She goes, 'Well, it's just – I've no hangover.'

'It was *morphine*!' I told her.

The next five minutes were pure howling with laughter down the phone. It was terrible and it was so funny.

'Never, ever tell a soul,' she made me promise.

Oops!! Well, at least I haven't named you.

* * *

I was in LA with my parents when I heard I had been nominated for the People of the Year award by an anonymous person who had seen me with one of the next generation of EB kids – Claudia – at the after-party of the Women's Mini Marathon. Claudia is twenty-one now, but at the time she was quite little. This person saw how I was encouraging her and thought it was worth recognising. I never got the person's name and so I never got to thank them.

The awards were being held in October and I wasn't allowed to tell anyone. *Not a soul.* I hung up the phone with my heart thumping in my chest and my hands shaking and immediately told my mother.

'You'll need a dress,' she said.

'So will you,' I replied.

Let's just put it this way, I didn't lick my love of fashion off the stones. My mother and her sisters have real energy for fashion – they love it, but they also love a bargain. I don't care about bargains, if I love something I will buy it straight away. Life's too short to be waiting for the sale.

Once we had the event to plan for, we started looking in LA

for the perfect dress. But that year, for some reason, everything was too casual. I like classy, timeless clothes, but the trend was playing against me. The more I looked, the more panicked I got.

'I can wear something I have,' I said. But Mom insisted we keep looking.

My girls' group chat had exploded with the news. (Yes, I know, I was supposed to keep quiet, but this dress disaster was serious and I needed them.)

'You know what?' Lynn said. 'I'm going to email a few designers and see if we can sort something nice.'

So she did. And the Dublin designer Deborah Veale was the first to reply, with a *YES* straight away; she even offered to close her shop for the afternoon so I could come in privately.

In LA I met up with my friend Gavin, who lives in Vegas. We met when he was doing *Jigs 'n' Reels* on RTÉ and he chose Debra Ireland as his charity. That's how we met – he was one of the dancers, in his twenties. Me being me, of course, I had a huge crush on him. My radar was really off though, as he later went off to America and married his lovely husband, Marcus.

We had gone to Vegas once as a family, but Gavin was away. We'd had a good time: we saw *The Lion King,* which was amazing, and the famous fountain, and we did have fun in the hotels and casinos, but the heat was too much. We couldn't stick it. Still I'd love to go back again – maybe someday.

I remember that time in LA, Gavin was pushing me along the boardwalk in my wheelchair when a woman skated past us on roller blades, looked at us as she passed and then skidded to a halt. She turned to look, skated again for a bit, and then stopped and skated back for a better look.

'What the hell was that?' Gavin said, in his lovely northern accent.

'Probably me,' I said.

'I don't think so,' he said.

We never figured out which one of us it was or what she was actually staring at. It might have been that she'd seen Gavin in Vegas. It might have been that she'd never seen anybody like me before, but either way, it was really funny. Her double take was so obvious.

America's really like that – people there are more open with their curiosity, they really go for it. The Irish would have tried to be more sneaky about that glance.

As soon as I got home from LA, I went in to see Deborah Veale. Her shop was on St Stephen's Green. I felt so important that day, she really gave me the 'Pretty Woman' experience – though without Richard Gere, unfortunately! I think we looked at every single dress. I probably tried on half of them. And in the end I chose a beautiful red ballgown with a sweetheart neckline and puffed shoulders.

I didn't expect it and I was delighted, but later I was told in secret that I had won. I kept that largely to myself, just telling Mom and Dad.

'I didn't expect to win,' I said to Mom, 'but I really wish the whole family could come.'

I wanted my family to be on the spot when they called out my name, so they would feel the same pride for me that I always did for them.

'I know, Emma,' she said, 'but it's June's wedding the same day.'

Awards night came. Debra Ireland had two tables, and all my friends were there. Except of course for my family. I wanted to be at June's wedding just as much as they wanted to be at my award ceremony, but it was just one of those clashes that cannot be helped.

We were in the hotel room, wondering what to do with ourselves – just waiting – when there was a knock at the door.

'Room service,' a familiar voice called. It was my cousin Aoife, coming to surprise me.

'I couldn't miss this,' she said and gave me a big hug. She told me the whole family were going to watch the TV during the wedding and root for me in spirit.

Gráinne Seoige was hosting. We had filmed a short piece beforehand at a barbecue with friends and family. They said it would be a small thing, but it turned into a whole segment. They played the video on the big screen, clips and voice-overs saying wonderful things about me – I was touched and embarrassed in equal measures.

When my name was called, Mom, wearing this gorgeous purple halter-style dress, pushed me up onto the stage. Ray D'Arcy presented my award. That was how I met Ray. We became firm friends that night and he even became an ambassador for Debra Ireland.

On stage Ray spoke about EB, how it affects people, and then said, 'We've got a very special fan of Emma's here tonight.'

The screen behind him lit up and there was Colin Farrell. 'Hi, Emma,' he said and waved through the screen. We hadn't met yet. This was the first time I had ever heard Colin say my name. My heart did backflips.

Unbeknownst to me, when the producers were looking for a celebrity to record a message for the winner, Jimmy said, 'What about Colin? He's already agreed to the dinner.'

Colin, of course, said yes. That's the first thing I love about him, he is so approachable, and Jimmy had told him all about me.

Then Colin said, 'Emma, since I can't be there to wear the

face off ya, I'm actually here wearing your face on a T-shirt.' And he was!

I burst out laughing. It was so *him*. That Dublin down-to-earth way about him that makes him the nation's darling.

On screen, he talked about me and my story, what I'd done, what I meant to people. The whole thing was surreal. I hadn't expected to win anything. I hadn't even expected to be nominated. And yet, here I was, in a designer dress, being called 'an inspiration' by a movie star.

People often call me that – an inspiration. Although, now that I think of it, there was one day I went into a Trócaire shop, and a woman working there kept calling me 'the celebrity'. She kept saying to other customers, 'Mind the celebrity!' or 'She's a celebrity, you know.' I was mortified.

But inspiration is a word I hear all the time, and sometimes I wonder if it's thrown around too easily. I don't identify with that word at all, although I do understand why it's used. To me, this work has never been about inspiring people.

When I am on TV, or at an event, or doing a challenge, all I want to do is to spread awareness about this condition and to help people understand it. That's not inspirational, not to me – I'm living with EB, it's not a choice I have.

That word inspirational can become a label to stick on people who live with something difficult; it's a catch-all that flattens you to one dimension. You become an inspiration and the word loses meaning. Your life takes that on and people see a positive.

There is no positive to living with EB.

I think there's a difference between being an inspiration and giving someone hope. Inspiration is what puts the drive in you to do something for yourself, hope is what comes *from* you, a quiet belief that things *can* get better, even when there's no evidence yet. Maybe inspiration makes you want to go on. But *hope* is the fuel that keeps you going on. I get the difference. I want people affected by EB to see me and to think, *If she can go to college, live independently, drive a car – maybe my child can too.*

That's what I want to do – give others hope. I don't want to inspire them to live better, or to be better, that's not my job. I want to represent EB and show other patients and families and the public that this awful condition exists; that we exist and we need help. We need hope.

I complain sometimes. All the time, if I am honest. Of course I do – I'm in pain. I live with EB. But I want people, especially those coming after me, to see that living with this *is* possible. I want to shout out to them, 'Look this way! I went to college. I've worked. I've lived on my own. I can drive.'

I want kids, and their parents, Claudia and Casey and all the little ones, to see me out in the world and think, *I can do that too*. That's the message. That's what matters.

Writing this really reminds me of Bobby. He and I used to talk about hope like it was something you could trade. Bobby's dream was to live on his own. Mine was to drive. We each had what the other wanted. It was like we had swapped hopes. That stuck with me. Maybe hope is something tradable, something tangible you can give another person.

That's what hope looks like to me: the passing of light, back and forth.

I believe this is what I'm meant to do. Hope is the reason I'm here. It's the reason I fought past a week, a month, a year and every year since. It's the reason I struggled and refused to lose my softness. Even when I was silenced. This is why.

I've found my voice now.

Hope is power.

22

Enchanted

The minute Colin Farrell sat down I knew I was going to like him.

The best way I can put this is he looks like a star and he walks like a star, but when Colin opens his mouth to talk, the Hollywood falls off him. That suave celebrity you see in movies and on the red carpet? In reality, he is a darling.

I'd spent weeks finding a dress for the fundraisers' dinner – red, gorgeous. I'd spent ages getting ready, full make-up, hair. I hadn't choked much in years, but I wasn't taking the chance of spluttering all over Colin Farrell, so I rang the hotel in advance and ordered plain mashed potatoes for my meal. I wanted to play it really safe and just have things I knew would definitely not cause any problems.

Everything was set.

But that didn't stop the bad weather that had been brewing for days, and before we knew it word was coming through that flights were being cancelled because of the snow.

Colin was in London, and word started to circulate that he might not make it at all.

'He has to!' I was thinking of all the women who had campaigned and raised extraordinary amounts. It would be so disappointing if he didn't get here.

If I had known Colin then like I do now, I wouldn't have worried. I think he would have swum the Irish Sea if he'd had to. I found out later that he was planning to get the ferry from Holyhead if his flight was cancelled.

The text came in: Colin had made it. The event was going ahead as planned. No panic.

We had to go by train as the snow was so deep at that point. It added a magic to the air.

When we arrived at the dinner, there was a buzz like I had never felt. Five women had raised thousands between them, and they each had a seat at the event, with one empty chair where Colin would sit beside them when he did the rounds. It was going to be wonderful.

'In between rounds,' Jimmy whispered, 'we have put his base chair next to you.'

My nerves went into overdrive; it felt like a flock of geese in my tummy, not butterflies. I couldn't wait for Colin to sit down in the empty seat next to mine.

We had to get a little lift up to the event, one of those with only room for two and a door you had to open yourself. The button, the man told us, had to stay pressed to make it go. Myself and Mom were so focused on that, that we forgot who we were going to meet. The door opened, and suddenly I was hugging a man in a big winter coat.

It was Colin. I'd hardly had time to take a breath when he was whipped away to meet other people. That was fine, I told myself, I'd see him at dinner when he sat beside me.

And the moment he did, well, it felt like I was his oldest friend in the world.

'Howyah,' he said, pulling his chair back and sitting down.

I was stunned. But I pulled myself together straight away.

'Hi, Colin,' I said.

'I'm starving, are you?' he said, as if we were siblings at the family table.

Suddenly I was. Actually being in his company, turns out I wasn't nervous at all. Thankfully the food came out right away.

Our meals went down in unison – his plate, my plate. *Uh-oh.* They had fancied up my mashed potatoes with chopped *raw* onion.

Even on my best day, raw is never an option. I called the waiter back before he got too far from me.

'I rang last week,' I said. 'I had pre-ordered mashed potatoes.'

'Those are mashed potatoes,' he said and pointed at the bowl.

I glanced sideways hoping Colin was chatting elsewhere. I didn't want to cause a fuss. But he was facing me and watching the interaction.

'Sorry,' I said, lowering my voice, 'it's just that there is onion in them and I can't ... I can't eat them ... could I get plain mashed potatoes please?'

The waiter hummed and hawed, staring at the plate and then back towards the kitchen.

'We don't really have any other ...' he said and trailed off mid-sentence. When I glanced to my right I saw Colin's face. He had a look on him that said, 'I dare you to say no to her.'

Colin is fun and so endearing, but he is also – from the core – a really decent and *good* human. And when he wants to be, fierce!

That look hit home. I think the waiter would have picked the onions out by hand after he saw it. He grabbed my bowl, ran off and came back about five minutes later with plain mashed potato.

I knew right there and then that I had just seen the foundations go down for a friendship that would see me through the rest of my life.

Colin and I kept in touch after that, by email and then text. From the start I always just wrote to him like I would any friend, filling him in on my life and asking questions about his. I've always been an open-book kind of person, and I treated our emails as though they were letters to a pen pal. He began to respond to me in the same way. We still write to one another a lot, and talk, like friends do, about deep and personal things.

Now, I would say Colin is one of my closest friends. He can trust me – that's the truth – and I can trust him. That is sacred to me. People always lean in and say, 'Give me the goss on Colin,' and I get the joke, I do. But there is nothing anyone could give me or say to me to get me to betray Colin's trust. I want to be a real friend to him, not because he is a celebrity, but because I genuinely think he is a great person – it's the same reason I choose all my friends. But with Colin's career skyrocketing, I know he has to be extra careful of his private life. I'm not even tempted to name-drop or show off our friendship, because that's something I never wanted from anyone – the glamour of their name or fame by proxy.

Our friendship grew from that moment with a bowl of mashed potato: one look that told me this guy had my back, and a feeling that I wanted to be friends for life with this sincere and funny human who stuck up for me over a handful of misplaced onions.

Even if Colin were a chimney sweep, I would feel that way.

23

A Place in this World

Killashee Hotel is a gorgeous venue in Naas. It's a historic building, now a hotel, set in its own grounds. Jimmy and I started meeting there for coffee sometimes, instead of me coming all the way to Dublin. We could do our usual putting heads together activity there, with nicer coffee for sure, and while we were there this one time in 2011, we met up with Conor, who was involved with Killashee.

'Killashee are planning a new garden,' Jimmy said, Conor nodding along, 'dedicated to Debra Ireland.'

I loved the idea; I thought it was a really beautiful sentiment and I said so.

'We want to bring you in,' Conor said, 'to work on the design and purpose of the space.'

I said immediately that I thought it could be a butterfly garden, a place where people with EB could come and sit in nature, safely, and enjoy watching butterflies as they fly from flower to flower. These little creatures represent the EB community in so many ways: they are as fragile as we are, they are as resilient as we are, and they are beautiful – just like we are. Butterflies represent Debra Ireland too, as their logo.

'Deal,' said Conor, 'a butterfly garden it is. The brainchild of Emma Fogarty.'

It was agreed we would build a butterfly garden, planting all the flowers that butterflies love.

'This is so special,' I said.

Conor went quiet for a moment and then he turned to me and said, 'Emma, how would you feel if we named the garden after you?'

I was so surprised, and I will admit my first emotion felt like guilt. There are so many people, so many children and adults with EB, and they each deserve a garden named for them. I felt really torn, but of course I wasn't going to reject this wonderful offer. I couldn't say no, I didn't say no. I loved it. It still means so much to me.

I popped down on and off as the garden was built, and I felt the same swell of pride each time. As the months went on and the work progressed, it looked more and more like a garden, and I watched this lovely space emerge in front of my eyes. The planting happened so quickly, and suddenly it was there and ready for people to visit.

When I arrived at Killashee for the opening there must have been 200 people waiting for me. My parents, my sister and my aunts were there, and there was a rake of my cousins and their children too. The Debra team, so many of our nursing friends from our EB clinic. Nurse Anne Sloane from James's Hospital even came. It was a great crowd. Ray D'Arcy was there – he had become our ambassador after the People of the Year Awards those few years earlier. Johnny Sexton was invited too, as our star ambassador, to open the garden with me.

I'd met Johnny at a photo call years previously, and we had become instant friends. On that first meeting, I went in with a plan: to tell him all about EB and to be as open and honest as I could. I wanted him to understand, not just what EB is, but what it means to live with it. The everyday. The emotional toll. The invisible stuff.

He listened. He asked questions. And he became my friend.

Kim told me later that Johnny hadn't been sure if he could be a Debra ambassador – a conflict with another charity, I think – but apparently after our chat, he changed his mind. She said he told her he did it because he met me. That floored me. It meant a lot.

So I was delighted to see Johnny at the opening of the garden.

'We're cutting the ribbon together,' he said, taking the handles of my chair to push me. As we turned to go down, the sun came out and the garden looked so inviting and lovely it took my breath away. This garden was for those who might need it – families, patients, carers, anyone can go in, close the little gate behind them and just be still, in a pocket of solace where you can let your worries drift for a while.

'I feel like I'm going to cry,' I whispered over my shoulder.

'Don't,' he whispered, 'you'll start me off.'

As we got closer, I noticed a sign on the gate that said, 'EMMA'S BUTTERFLY GARDEN'.

'Oh wow, Emma, look,' Mom said, but I couldn't reply. A whole lifetime of emotion was stuck in my throat. I just waved my hand and held back the tears. I can't describe it, the feeling in that moment – like I was giving something back to the community that had held me up for so long.

Johnny and I each held a handle each of the big scissors and attempted to cut the ribbon, but either the angle was wrong or the scissors were blunt, because they just went back and forth and didn't even crease the thing!

Johnny started looking at me with this face that said, 'What will we do?'

We both got the giggles.

'Help me out here, will ya?' I said. My shoulders were shaking so much from laughing it was making the whole thing worse.

We swapped the scissors around, went for another angle and seemed to make some progress.

We eventually got through the ribbon, but by then everyone was laughing along with us. There was such joy in the air, and there was a big cheer when we finally cut it.

Once that was done, the garden was open. I thought I would find a nice place to sit in the hotel and welcome people to the reception, but ... nope. I was hurried upstairs with Johnny to give interviews on the phone. For the next hour or two it was just me and Johnny sitting in a hallway passing two phones back and forth.

'Hi, it's Johnny.'

'Hi, it's Emma.'

We spoke to the *Mirror*, the *Star*, the *Indo*. Mad, but really brilliant. By the time we were finished everyone was having a great time. The atmosphere was gorgeous. People just chatting, eating, being together.

'Have you your speech ready?' I said to Johnny as we rounded the door.

His face fell.

'Am I ... nobody told me ...'

'I'm joking!' I said, because I *was*.

We went in and mingled, and then came the speeches. Ray told a lovely story about how we met. Then the microphone was passed to Jimmy.

Suddenly Jimmy called out to Johnny to say a few words.

I'll never forget it. I think I was more surprised than Johnny.

He turned to me as he walked up to the stage and gave me a look that said, *you're for it!*

'I didn't know!' I said, but he didn't believe me.

I'm great friends with Johnny. I can say that. I've visited his home in 2018 and met his family. I loved being in his house. It's lived in, like a real home – evidence of his children and his life everywhere. When we were there, he brought his medals down and talked about each one.

'Which one can I have?' I said. They were all so heavy.

Johnny was in the running for rugby player of the year that year, and I remember standing out at the car just before I went home saying to him, 'You've got this! This is yours for the taking.'

Later that year he won 'World Player of the Year'. I was so happy when I found out.

Johnny is one of Ireland's greatest people, I'm so proud of him. He never fails to support Debra whenever he can. He's stayed involved, shown up when it mattered, and lent his voice to our cause. And that's all I ever really want – for people to see us. To really see us. Not just the surface, not just the hardship, but the strength too. And, of course, the hope.

I will always visit the little butterfly garden at Killashee. If you see me there, come up and say hello. There's a little treasure trail for kids too, with letters hidden around to make up a word. The hotel put it all together beautifully. I love showing it to people. I'm really proud of it.

If you ever can, pop in to see it. You don't have to be a guest of the hotel; you can just go and take a moment.

* * *

Coming up to my thirtieth, I decided to try driving again. I was more cautious this time, more anxious maybe – but also more determined. I knew the freedom driving had to offer – an ability to go where I pleased, to move without waiting, to go places without planning, on a whim.

That mattered more than ever.

This time, I had the right car and that changed everything. Through Debra Ireland, Nissan had surprised me with a specially adapted car. I was able to use this car for a year, and if I wanted to buy it after that I could. It was a huge boost.

I still remember how it felt, climbing into the driver's seat and preparing to move forward for the first time. It was terrifying, yes, but exhilarating too. Like I was reclaiming something I hadn't even realised had been taken.

On the day of the test, I shook all the way through. I don't remember most of it – just how tightly I was holding myself together. I did my best. Was I nervous? God, yes. Did I do well? Hmmm ... I think the tester passed me out of sheer shock that we both made it back alive.

I could hardly believe it when he handed me the pink cert, and I don't think he quite could either.

Maybe he saw what it meant to me to be able to drive. Maybe that was enough to ignore me taking corners like wing mirrors weren't a thing.

Either way, I had a licence now.

I'll never forget the moment I turned the key with my licence in my handbag on the floor beside me – I was truly moving under my own steam again.

* * *

A few weeks before that same birthday we had been at the Kerry Challenge in Dingle: me, Kim, Caitriona and Lynn. The four of us don't get to see each other as much as we did in our twenties. Except for Kim, their careers have moved on from Debra Ireland, although they are still all involved on a personal level. But we always come together at events and especially when there's something to celebrate.

'Let's get really dressed up tonight,' Lynn suggested for our last night, 'and do something nice.' So I got my hair done, wore make-up and a pretty dress. I even wore fake eyelashes for the first (and last) time in my life.

'Wooo,' said Kim, as we got into the car, 'you look fab.'

'So do you!' I told her. It was nice to get dolled up.

I remember Kim was driving me to meet the girls when – even though there was no traffic – she slowed the car and beeped the horn really loudly. Suddenly little Casey's grandad, who I knew, jumped out from behind a parked car dressed as a Mario Brother.

'What is he doing?' I said, as 'Mario' gestured us into the car park of the pub nearby.

It took me a minute to realise this show was for me. But the minute I walked inside I knew what was going on. Everyone I knew jumped out and yelled, 'Happy Birthday, Emma!'

The girls had organised a pre-birthday, unofficial birthday do – a huge surprise party in the beer garden of a pub in Dingle. I worried for a moment that they had forgotten I already had a party planned.

'That's your official thirtieth,' Kim said, 'this is your unofficial thirtieth.'

Nearly everyone I knew was there, and the party had the full works. There was a cake, there was a DJ, there was a photographer, Richie, and I even gave a speech.

'I am the fourth person with EB to reach thirty,' I said. It made me so happy to say that out loud, but it also made my heart ache for Bobby. My birthday would always be his anniversary – it was already five years since he had passed away. I wished he was there smiling back at me.

The cake they brought out was shaped like a handbag, handles and all. It was gorgeous. But I was having a problem. The fake lashes were hard to wear. My God. I tried to persevere, but my eyes watered so much that eventually Kim just pulled them off. I remember when she said she was going to, we both looked at each other, knowing what my skin was like – this could make my night or break it.

Neither of us fancied a trip to the hospital because I had no eyelids.

'How strong is the glue?' I said. 'Do you think it'll tear my eyelid off?'

'Only one way to find out,' she said as we grimaced at each other, held our breath and she pulled the first one away. I didn't feel a thing!

Once they were gone, I could really relax.

I had my 'official' party the following week in Durrow, County Laois. Everyone was there, including Bobby's family, all squashed into an old pub called Bob's Bar. The place was rammed. Lynn was in America but she FaceTimed us. I could only wave and so could she – the place was so loud we couldn't hear each other.

Later, Bobby's family pulled me out for a dance because 'Thriller' came on. As I swayed in my wheelchair and they danced around me, I missed Bobby so much, but it wasn't with sadness, it was with a feeling of light.

A feeling of, *he would have loved this*.

24

Bad Blood

Imagine being dependent on someone else if you want to live independently. Imagine always having to rely on another adult for every single thing, from using the bathroom, to grabbing a coffee, to going to the shops, to meeting a friend. I can't do any of those common things – let alone anything else – without help. Sometimes that help is my mother, sometimes it's my sister or an aunt or a cousin, but mostly it's one of my personal assistants. They are with me all day as I live my life. Can you even imagine that?

Over the years, I've worked with numerous personal assistants. Most of those relationships have been good – some even great. But there have also been times when things have been less positive.

Often, it would start well, but then slowly, something would shift. I could never put my finger on why, but things would just start to feel tighter. Heavier. And eventually, something between us would break.

In one case, I began to notice small things: my PA would arrive late, leave early, or change plans at the last minute. There were days off without much warning. I'd find myself having to cancel coffee with friends, throw out tickets for events I couldn't attend, or watch my mother or sister scramble to fill the gap.

Sometimes, when she did show up, she would leave early, with little notice.

'I won't be in next week at all,' one told me on a Friday when she was driving me home. I was stunned. I had a couple of things coming up, including a medical appointment. I couldn't go by myself, and I knew my mom was not able to step in this time.

'But I need you to come in,' I said, 'I have that appointment. Mom is busy.'

'Well,' she said, 'I'm taking the week.'

I would try to explain that I needed consistency. I needed to know I could make plans and keep them. That I could rely on the system. I didn't feel heard.

Things got so bad that my mom decided to try talking to that PA. I don't know if you've ever met my mother, but she is really gentle. I've rarely heard a bad word escape her lips, she is such a lady. So you can imagine how hurt I felt when she came back from this talk really upset.

Eventually, I stopped making fixed plans. 'Let me check with my PA,' became my default answer. I felt I could no longer shape my life around what I wanted to do. I was even told on one occasion that I was being ungrateful! That's not independence.

I mean, look, the role of a PA is pretty clear. They are there to enable independence. Mine, not theirs. Maybe that PA was burned out, maybe her private life was hard at that time, but those are explanations, not excuses. There is no excuse. The leader–PA relationship has to be a good fit. If it's not, it chips away at you. You feel powerless. And for someone as vulnerable as I am, that kind of environment is unbearable. When it's difficult, it leaves a mark. And I think it matters that this is said.

The truth is, when you rely on someone every day to help

you live, when it's not working it doesn't just inconvenience you. It breaks you. You can't just walk away. You're reliant. And they know it. That imbalance can be dangerous. When you live with a condition like mine, the wrong person in that role is not just a hassle. It's a threat to your peace and your sense of self.

Yes, I want to get on with my PA, and yes, I want to be flexible and understanding, but there is a real difference between being understanding and being a doormat. Being independent means having the right to make and keep plans. It means having space for joy, spontaneity and the ordinary things that make life full. Some people think missing a coffee date or rescheduling a shopping trip is no big deal. Yet able-bodied people don't have to, so we shouldn't have to either. It's not frivolous to be independent. It's not selfish to want control over your own life. It's a human right.

The right person respects you. They enable your choices. Just like Georgina Herlihy does.

* * *

'What's on the schedule?' Georgina Herlihy said when she walked in that first time.

'I've no plans,' I said.

She put her hands on her hips.

'Alright so,' she said, 'what do you fancy doing?'

'I don't mind,' I said.

'Ah, Jaysus,' Georgina said, with a wink, 'do I have to organise everything round here?'

That sudden warmth (yes, that is the Irish being loving, believe it or not) was a joy.

'I'd love to go for a coffee,' I suggested.

'Right,' she said, and set about sorting me to get into the car.

Once she was assigned to me, George went up to be trained in St James's Hospital – first the theory, then the practice on me. She learned carefully and she's excellent. At first, she did my bandages on her own, but as my condition deteriorated, we needed help. On Fridays, she works with my local public health nurse. On Tuesdays, Thursdays and Saturdays, she works with agency nurses who are fully trained.

Another time in that first week, George asked me what I fancied doing one day. I said I didn't have any plans.

She shook her head. 'Let's go somewhere.'

'Sure,' I said, 'but where will we go?'

'I'll surprise you,' she said and put my chair into the car.

The next thing we pulled in at a forest walk.

'I don't know, Georgina,' I said, as we headed off, 'the path looks a bit rough.'

'You'll be grand,' she said.

Rough? I had no idea. Right around the corner the path went from gravel to a wooden slatted walkway that stretched over a bog.

'Georgina!' I yelled, but she just pushed me straight onto it. 'I'll fall out!' I tried to look over my shoulder, but she was bent over with the effort it was taking to push my chair along this rickety walkway.

'You won't,' she said, and there was fun in her voice, 'and if you do, I'll pick you up and put you back in.'

Well, I burst out laughing and held on as I bounced from plank to plank along the bog walk. I was … not terrified … more *thrilled* in the way I was on the rides in Alton Towers, or on the pony I rode, or on my bike going downhill. I was scared, but in the way you get when you're stepping out of your comfort zone.

Yes, this could end with wounds, but so could *anything*. In that moment I knew George was a good one.

I will never forget the first birthday I had with George. Early on, when we had been getting to know each other, I'd mentioned that I had never been on a girly weekend. It was an offhand comment, a response to George talking about something like that. But, in typical George fashion, she surprised me with a night away in a hotel with my closest girlfriends on my birthday. I was really touched.

For the last six years, George has been my full-time PA, but honestly, that title doesn't come close to capturing what she means to me. We like the same things: music, shopping, going to the cinema. The different interests we have are also things we can talk over. We do the same things friends do, and over time that's exactly what we became – true friends.

PAs are there to help you live your life, get out and about, support you during the day, things like that. George and I used to call it a 'PA-ship' instead of a friendship, because the role is about enabling independence. George not only enables me to be independent, she pushes me to be more independent. I'm lucky. We're a team. We've built a relationship on trust, understanding and good craic.

George is fiercely protective. And when you live with something like EB, having that in your corner makes a world of difference.

In everyday life, she knows my cues. We use 'eyesight language' where a glance between us is enough. She can tell when I'm uncomfortable in a room full of people or when I'm unsure of something. At the dentist, she advocates when I'm too shy. I've known my dentist since he was a student, and now he's senior staff in a teaching hospital. I trust him. I don't trust the students who don't know EB. So George will step in: 'She feels comfortable with you. She'd prefer if you did the treatment.' That kind of backup is everything.

We even have our own little traditions.

At the Kerry Challenge every year, on the Saturday night there's a band and dancing. A few years ago, George grabbed my hand when a slow song came on and said, 'Come on, we're doing the slow set.' Now it's our tradition – just the two of us on the dance floor, swaying, people staring or not. It doesn't matter. We just do it.

Georgina Herlihy is my personal assistant, but she is also one of my closest friends.

Georgina Herlihy has never let me down. *Never*. She pushes me when I doubt myself.

I remember saying to her once, half-joking, that I'd love to write a book someday, but everyone would just laugh and say it was too depressing.

She looked at me for a second or two.

'Yes, your life is hard,' she said, 'but you've also had a good life. You've done amazing things. Write the book, Emma.'

That's George. She sees the whole of me.

25

Tears in Heaven

Living with EB isn't just about managing pain – though God knows, that's a battle. It's also about living with loss. Over and over again. It's about falling in love with people who are fighting the same battle as you – and then losing them. Too young, too suddenly, and far too often.

I'd known Liam from a baby. I knew him all his short life. The minute I met him, at Bobby's casino night, I fell in love.

Bobby had been gone for seven years when we lost Liam too.

* * *

I didn't see Liam and his family often – they lived in Monaghan and it wasn't easy for me to travel. But I always knew how he was getting on. I'd see him at Debra Ireland events and he'd always be the same little boy, sweet and gentle. He had so much grace for someone so young and in such pain. Watching him grow up was like watching a little light shine through everything. At the last Debra Christmas party, he looked great. Happy out, playing on his iPad, full of life.

Then came an event at Barretstown in September 2016. I knew he'd be there, and I was looking forward to see him. I was sitting with Claudia, and when Liam and I spotted each other, his whole face lit up. His mom, grandparents – even his great-grandparents – were there. I'd gotten to know his family over the years, and they are the warmest, most dedicated people. Like my own, they gave *everything* for their child.

I spent a while that day with Liam, chatting about bandages, football, arts and crafts. He told me he supported Liverpool and that he'd even tried playing football. I nearly fell off my chair laughing when he told me that – but honestly, I wasn't surprised. That fighting spirit was so *him*. He lived more fully in his few short years than some people do in decades.

As the day wound down, I didn't want to leave. If I'd known it was the last time I'd see him, I never would have. We took a photo, and I asked him the big question this time: 'Liam, will you be my future husband?' (Just like I'd been asked by an older EB patient, Aaron, all those years ago). Liam looked at me and said, 'Maybe!'

I burst out laughing. That little spark of innocence, humour and love – it just killed me. I adored him.

Three weeks later, the worst news came.

It was a Friday night when Jimmy from Debra called to say Liam had become very unwell, very suddenly. I didn't believe it. I told myself, *It's Liam, he's strong, he'll be okay.* I clung to that hope.

But the next night my phone beeped. I couldn't look. My mom read it for me, and I knew from her face. My heart broke there and then.

There are no words for this kind of grief. Nothing prepares you for it. I couldn't eat. I couldn't sleep. All I did was cry. EB is so unfair. Liam was a little boy. If I could have taken his place, I would have.

The funeral was two days later. I was dreading it. How do you face a family that's lost a child? What can you possibly say? The church was packed. And I have to say, seeing that little white coffin on the altar shattered us all.

We went to the graveside. His grandmother hugged me, sobbing. Just sobbing. 'He's at peace now,' I said. 'It's going to be okay.'

But it wasn't okay. It was wrong. His mother was so young. Seeing her say goodbye broke everyone.

There is this bond between us all – unspoken, but deep. When one of us goes, it's never just one. And honestly, deep down, when something like this happens, I am *scared*. Liam had been doing so well. He was happy. And then ... gone. Just like that. EB doesn't give warnings. It doesn't play fair.

I've written a lot about pain. But nothing – *nothing* – comes close to describing this kind of heartbreak. I've known so many people with EB, I've lost so many too. I've loved them, laughed with them, mourned them. I carry each one of them with me.

Liam will always be something special. I feel so lucky to have had him in my life, even just for a while. His smile, his kindness, that cheeky little 'maybe' – they'll stay with me forever.

26

The Climb

My life changed completely in 2019 and I was left feeling like fate split it in two. The before I barely remember, and the after I'm still learning how to live with.

Yet again, my little foot had another wound, this time on the ankle. None of us had ever before seen a wound heal the way this one was doing.

I feel like I need to reiterate that there are wounds all over my body, constantly. Eighty per cent of my body is a wound. So, maybe you can imagine how it is, trying to keep an eye on what is good healing and figure out what is unusual. Wounds go through stages: sometimes they dry out a bit, scab over, go crusty, then that falls off and new skin is underneath. But most of the time we just have to manage the wound and try to heal it with antibiotic creams or steroid creams. I use a birch tree cream as well too. That cycle is my whole body all the time but at different stages. So, often times we really aren't sure if something is okay or ominous.

Something else I need to establish again, though I know I've mentioned it before, is that I hate going to hospital. I will resist until the last minute because it always means weeks of bed rest, and I hate that too. In a subconscious way I feel maybe like it's wasting my precious time to be in there, even though that thought is definitely counter-productive. But I will always, *always* take the wait-and-see approach.

A debate erupted.

'I'm not happy with that,' Georgina, my mom, the nurses, someone would say every bandage change.

'I'll give it a week,' I'd say.

They attempted to clean it out with a soft sponge, but it felt like a Brillo pad and I had to ask them to stop.

Eventually, I had to admit defeat. Especially when black spots appeared. The test in June was all clear, then another test in October was not.

To nobody's surprise it was cancer. Squamous cell carcinoma. The worst kind. I thought about Bobby.

Now the debate really began.

Should we try surgery on the ankle to save it or just go straight to worst-case scenario and amputate my leg? Squamous cell carcinoma is voracious once it gets in. We could take a chance and go through surgery and hope – or we could amputate.

In the end, the doctors made the call. 'We just can't guarantee we will get it all,' they said.

'Okay,' I said.

I could not get my thoughts to process. Fear overwhelmed me. I don't think I really fully understood what I was telling them to do. But the surgeons, George and my parents were all looking anxious, and once I gave my final answer, they agreed with me immediately.

The surgery was scheduled so quickly I think that frightened me more than the diagnosis.

I was brought into hospital the day before, on a Wednesday. Everyone came up to be with me: Daddy, Mom, Catherine, George.

I was a wreck.

'I'm so nervous,' I whispered to Mom.

'What's getting to you?' she whispered back. 'Is it surgery nerves or that you're worried about your leg?'

'I don't know,' I said. She sat on the edge of the bed and stroked my hair.

The anaesthetist came in.

'Emma,' he said, 'we are going to be doing this surgery with an epidural.'

There was a collective gasp, but I was sure I had misunderstood.

'Wait,' I said, 'do you mean I'll be awake?'

He nodded slowly, 'Yes.'

Everyone else in the room stood up.

'Why?' my mother said.

The reason, he told us, is because if you are fully unconscious when having an amputation, your brain won't register the limb being removed, and later you can have phantom pain. For example, you'll feel itching in a foot that's not there. That still happens sometimes anyway, but the theory is that keeping you awake reduces the intensity.

I don't know. It seemed so barbaric.

They gave me a website link so I could read about the procedure, but I couldn't bring myself to look at it. I didn't want to know the details. I didn't want to see diagrams or explanations. I just wanted time. Not to accept it – because how do you ever accept that? I wanted space to sit with it. I wanted to be by myself to deal with this. To get the thought into my head properly: *Tomorrow, I'll wake up and they will saw off my leg.*

George and Dad left early, around eight, but Mom and Catherine stayed.

I remember it was around twelve o'clock and I wanted to say, 'I just need you to go away.' But I couldn't say it out loud. As if she read my mind, Mom said, 'I'm staying with you for as long as I can.'

'No, you go,' I said. 'I'm only going to fall asleep soon, I'm fine.'

But she insisted. 'I'm going to stay until you fall asleep.' I was thinking, *How am I supposed to fall asleep with you sitting silently, just staring at me?*

Maybe she worried I'd flap if I was left alone. But the truth is, I was flapping anyway. If I had cried, it might actually have done me good, it might have let something out of my system. But I couldn't.

I needed to sleep. I couldn't do that either.

It got to a point where I had to ask for a sleeping tablet. Thankfully, they gave me one. I drifted off eventually, and, at some point, I heard a rustle of people leaving. I was already too far gone to react or say anything, even though, when it came to it, I had changed my mind. But I couldn't call them back or cry or say, 'Don't go.'

The next morning came and I was fourth in line for surgery. I didn't want to be alone at that point. I wanted someone with me all the time.

How can this be happening?

The doctor handling the amputation was a plastic surgeon. Apparently, that's who deals with this kind of operation.

And, of course, because I have EB, surgery is never straightforward. Everything has to be handled differently – carefully.

I asked for something to relax me, but they didn't give me anything. I kept saying to everyone, 'Please stay with me. Don't leave me. Just don't leave me.'

The doctor came around that morning.

'You're actually now number three on the list.' She explained that she'd had to bump someone else because they'd smoked after being told not to.

'So don't smoke,' she said and pointed a finger. It was funny, but I couldn't laugh. This was so serious. *My leg.*

The waiting started. That feeling settled in – the one where you're torn between, *Oh God, I never want them to come*, and *Oh God, I really want them to come now.* My whole body was trembling from top to bottom.

'Are you cold?' George asked and pulled up the blanket. But I wasn't, I was just so nervous. I remember thinking, *I'm about to lose my leg and I'll be awake for it. This is a piece of me. How can I go through this awake?*

It felt like I went into that hospital room as Emma, and I was going to come out as someone else. A completely different person.

Eventually, the porter came to bring me down to theatre. Everyone was around me, hugging me, kissing me. George was holding my hand. What I didn't know until afterwards was that a leader she had worked with before me had passed away that same day and that she got the message just before I was wheeled down for surgery.

Mom noticed something in her expression and asked her if she was okay. George just said, 'I'm grand,' put on her game face and kept walking beside me.

Then it was all corridors and white lights above me, flicking past. I was on the trolley, being wheeled along, and all I could think was, *Why is this happening to me?*

I'd seen that view a thousand times, but it felt different this time.

Mom was near my head, just holding my hand, a quiet force of safety. Catherine had my other hand. George was down near my leg with her hand on me, as if to subconsciously say, 'You can take her when I say you can.'

I was just lying there, tears streaming. I couldn't stop.

I remember thinking, *This is it. This is the moment my life changes forever.*

There was no going back.

You can't fix this with physio.

You can't un-lose a leg.

Even though I'd been using a wheelchair for years, I'd still had that hope. That someday, somehow, with the right physio or surgery or miracle, I'd get to stand again. Even just once. I always thought, *Maybe someday.*

But this … *this* was the end of it. There's no standing after this. There's no prosthetic either – believe me, we tried. It's all gone. The hope is gone. I will never stand up by myself ever again. A thought passed through my mind just then: *I will never stand beside Catherine as a maid of honour.*

They brought me into theatre, even though I was totally freaking out. I could see the doctors along the corridor, all the ones who knew me, saying their hellos, giving a nod. It felt like a funeral procession. *This is really happening.*

Every part of me was saying, *I can't do this. I can't do this.* But the theatre staff were ready, and then Mom and Catherine gave me a kiss, and George kissed my fingertips. I started repeating, over and over, 'No, please. No. I can't.'

The last thing I saw as I went through the doors was my mother. I reached out for her.

And the last thing I said – God help me – was, 'Mom, I'm sorry.'

I didn't even mean to say it. It just came out. I knew in that moment my life was being destroyed, but so was hers. I was going to be less able, more dependent. My family were going to have to carry even more of me.

That's what I meant by it. That's why I said I was sorry.

When we got inside the room I couldn't believe it. There was Christina, my EB nurse, and there was Suzi, Bobby's sister. Having her there in the theatre brought me real, deep comfort. She knew. She *knew* what it meant to go through this. She was the perfect person to be there. Suzi understood.

Christina came over and said, 'Emma, I want to put earphones in your ears now, is that okay?' And I said, 'Yeah.' She asked what I wanted to listen to, offered me a few options. *What music do I want to hear while I'm losing my leg?*

I think I told her to put on an Ed Sheeran album, but I don't remember the music. I don't remember hearing anything at all. I know it happened, but it's a blank.

There was a moment in the theatre when the young anaesthetist was trying to get me into position for the epidural. I'm so fragile. I remember him trying to manoeuvre me, telling me he needed me to move my shoulder. They were injecting things into the cannula every two minutes – stuff to calm me, I suppose. I remember asking, 'What are you putting into me? Please, tell me what you're giving me.'

But I didn't get an answer.

All I remember was this doctor saying, 'I just need your shoulder, Emma,' and then nothing after that.

What they gave me was a strong sedative, like an amnesia drug. You stay awake, you talk, you look people in the eye, you carry on the conversation, but when that wears off, it's all gone. You have no memory of what happened. My last memory of the theatre is that line from the anaesthetist, and when my memories kick in again, I'm in recovery.

Even though I don't remember being in that room, I *was*. I was present. I saw the team amputate my leg. I heard it. I saw it. Somewhere, deep in my mind where I can't find it, I went through all of it.

The first thing I remember again is that I'm holding Christina's finger. Just one finger, gently. I don't know why or how. But that's what I was doing.

And then the first thing I said – I'll never forget it – was, 'The pain in my foot is gone, Christina.'

I didn't say, 'Is it gone?' I didn't say, 'Did they do it?' I said, 'The pain is gone.'

The foot pain I had lived with my whole life was gone. I wasn't relieved exactly. It was just a fact.

I'd had so many surgeries at that point that the recovery nurses knew me. One by one, they were coming up and saying, 'Hi, Emma, how are you? Do you know me?'

And whether I did or didn't, it didn't matter. I was floating on strong medication, chatting away like nothing had happened.

Eventually they brought me back to my room. I was still out of it on morphine, and I think I said 'Hi!' to everyone as I went along the hospital corridor like I was arriving at a party.

When I came around the door of my room to my red-eyed and grief-stricken reception party, I was so cheery I think it shocked them all into better spirits.

'Hiya, I'm back,' I said and I was definitely waving.

Later, Mom said to Suzi, 'It's just so final.'

And I repeated that: 'It's just so final.'

It's not something you can absorb straight away, that sort of loss. You say the words, but they don't land yet. Not fully.

With EB, we live with wounds, with pain, with constant damage to our bodies, but it always blisters, always bleeds, always hurts. And yet this ... this was different. This was *saving* me. The damage had gone too far. It was this or not being here. This amputation was going to save my life. So what was I crying for?

Well, having both legs had given me some independence, even in the wheelchair. I could use my feet to scoot the chair a bit, get myself to the bathroom, transfer myself from bed to chair to the car to a seat at a table – even if it wasn't easy, it was possible.

And then there's something people don't talk about enough – the feeling of your leg. Just the presence of it. That mattered too. This was part of me, even if it gave me trouble, even if it didn't work. It was me.

Right after the surgery the doctor came to see me.

'There was a second area of cancer, Emma,' she said. 'Unfortunately it was completely independent ... on the sole of your foot. We took it off, but the reality is that it could come back in two years.'

Just like that. She stood there for a moment, but I had nothing to say. What could I say? Thanks for that, you cut off my leg and it might be for nothing. What was the point?

I remember thinking, *It's over for me. I'm going downhill.*

When I had my first moment alone with my people, when the room had settled, the doctor had dropped her bomb, and the nurses had gone, Mom walked over.

'Right,' she said, 'well I want to look at it.'

I remember where everyone was. Dad was sitting on my right. George was on my left. Catherine was just behind Mom.

'Please don't let me see it,' I said. 'Please don't show me.'

So Mom lifted the sheet and looked really sad.

I knew it was done, but I wasn't ready to see it for myself. Not yet.

Afterwards, I had horrific night terrors, where a man was chasing me with a hatchet. In the dream I'd always be with my girls – Kim, Lynn and Caitriona – but he would only run after me. I can still see him. That dream burned into my brain. Nurses would come in to find me asleep, sweating through the sheets, or waking up shouting for help. So they put a nurse in to sit with me at night. Then I would wake up relieved in one way but still terrified because my leg was gone.

I didn't feel like myself any more. Definitely not. I remember thinking, *I'm not Emma. Emma had two legs.*

The Emma I was before – she was gone. Her confidence, her spark, the part of her that felt whole. All of it.

27

Out of the Woods

So what happened to my leg?

They took it. Checked it. Examined everything.

Then they gave me two options. One was to take the leg and have it buried. But I couldn't. I just couldn't imagine putting my own foot into a casket and down into the ground. That's a part of me. My body. My life.

It felt too strange. Too final. But, at the same time, so did the other option: incinerating it.

It's such a weird concept, having a part of yourself turned to smoke. A piece of you just gone. If I reached down now and put my hand where my foot should be ... it's nowhere. It's not here. It's not anywhere. It's just gone.

After all of that, losing my leg, the night terrors, the grief, the horror and pain, I still had to wake up the next day, like I wake up every day, and do a bandage change.

No matter what, no matter that Bobby had passed away. No matter if I was told I had cancer. No matter if I was sick. No matter if I had my leg sawn off while I was awake. I still had to get up and do my bandages.

No reprieve.

After the surgery, everything had to be done lying down. My shoulders, my back, everything. And when I say I was in pain, I mean I was screaming. Screaming in pain. They'd left the epidural line in and I couldn't move my leg. It felt like a massive rock was pressing down on it. No matter what I did, I couldn't lift it.

I remember them pulling me around the bed to adjust my position so they could wrap well, and I was screaming so loudly that one of the nurses literally ran out of the room to find the doctor from the pain service. He came up within ten minutes and prescribed me extra medication straight away.

Clearly there'd been a breakdown in communication between hospital departments, because a few minutes after they left, Joanne came in – a physiotherapist I'd known for years – not knowing what I'd just been through, and wanting me to get out of the bed.

'No.' I couldn't even look at her. 'No way.'

'Okay,' she agreed, 'I won't make you do anything, but could you try to lift your leg a little?'

So I tried, but I turned into a ball of sweat. I couldn't lift it even slightly. It felt like I was trying to lift a rock with my hip.

I thought, *Is this it now? Is this what my life is going to be?*

Then came the first full bandage change of the new leg – the little leg. Christina and the nurses were planning to do that on the Monday. I couldn't avoid it any more. I would have to see my leg.

Mom, Catherine and George were there when I realised.

'I need you here,' I told them, 'when I look at it for the first time. I need one of you to come.'

They were all wrecked. We all were. Everyone was emotionally and physically drained. But they were there when Christina removed the bandage.

My reaction surprised us all. I screamed and screamed like I had in my nightmares.

'Put it back!' I sobbed. 'Just put it back.'

It felt like I was being pulled out of reality seeing what was left – it broke something in me. Maybe it was my heart. It felt that way. I don't think that has ever healed.

The physios were really trying to get me moving. They had this kind of mock car set-up in the hospital – just a passenger seat, nothing more, which they used to train people with disabilities how to get in and out of a real car. They were trying to figure out if I could do it – how I'd manage when the time came.

I'd just been told I was not going to outrun cancer, and now they wanted me to climb into a pretend car. It felt like a joke, and it was painful and awkward and overwhelming.

I don't want to do this.

Something in me just shut down. I went silent. I couldn't speak. The physio was asking, 'Are you okay?' and I couldn't respond.

I was totally shut off. It was like a switch had flipped. I was exhausted. Physically, mentally, emotionally – just *done.*

* * *

One evening the door of my room opened and my aunt Angela came in clutching a plastic bag to her chest. I was happy to see her, I always was, but I was so low. My leg still felt like a rock was pressing on it, and so did my soul, as if I was being pulled under by the weight of everything I'd been through.

'That bag is going to rip,' I said. I could see that whatever was in it was heavy.

'Emma,' Angela whispered, as she came close and put the

plastic bag carefully down on the bed, 'I know you're struggling, so my neighbour let me bring something up to you, something special.'

She patted the bag, then leaned in. 'Emma, I have Padre Pio's glove with me,' she said. 'I brought it for you.'

She reached into the bag and pulled out Padre Pio's relic. 'It has to go to Mayo tonight,' she told me, 'but they've allowed it to do a detour.'

I looked at the glove – brown, fingerless and woollen – it seemed very normal. It was worn and there were holes in it. The case it was in was held together with layers of tape, probably from years of being passed around and held by the sick and the weary.

I held the relic while Angela took out a small prayer she had written and said it out loud. She put it on my leg, my heart and even touched it to my head. And that was it. She packed the relic back up. She hadn't even taken her coat off, the visit was so fast.

Angela told me to pray and go to sleep, which I did.

When I woke up the next morning the physio came in. 'Can we try again, Emma?' she said.

I sat up a bit and took a breath and tried. The rock feeling was gone. I knew then that I'd been part of another miracle.

That was six years ago this November.

* * *

After a few weeks, I got to go home.

The physios had trained George, Mom, Catherine and Dad how to manage me. It was a new world for everyone because up to that point I'd always been able to transfer myself. Now I was not just an amputee who needed assistance, but one so fragile you can't really lift her without tearing her skin.

With the four of them doing what they had been taught, I managed to get out of the car, into the house and into bed.

Later, I needed to go to the toilet. It took *forty* minutes with three people helping. It wasn't that it went wrong. It just wasn't easy. Training is one thing, but it's not the same when you're actually doing it, with your real body, in real pain. I was in agony with EB and couldn't take any weight on what was left of my leg. And to be honest, my emotions were so intense I couldn't find the grit to bear any of it. I couldn't catch my breath and I started sobbing like a new baby does when it's at the end of its tether. *This is it now. This is my life.*

'Did we hurt you?' Mom said.

I couldn't look at her. 'I can't do this,' I said, 'I can't do this.'

And I meant it.

I just could not see a life where people had to help me to the toilet every time, where the simplest move was going to take forty minutes. I wanted to rewind. I really did.

I will be totally honest here – I was also really, really embarrassed. That was an over-riding emotion. I had already spent my life being stared at and commented on. It's hard enough with EB. Now I was an amputee. Now there was another part of me that people could stare at and whisper about.

So right then and there I shut down, went inside myself, all the way, to the darkest side humans have. I wouldn't see anyone, I wouldn't talk. I was in pain and I acted like it, hiding away.

Is this confusing? Hadn't I just been spared death with this operation? I knew that. But I felt so *injured*. That is the only way to describe it. Of all the wounds I had had in my life, this emotional wound was the worst pain I had ever felt.

I hadn't lost my leg; I had lost Emma.

I didn't know who I was.

Nobody could get through to me.

Then Colin FaceTimed.

'How's the head?' he asked.

He was the first person to ask that question. Maybe it was because he was farthest away. Maybe the people close to me were as lost as I was and didn't ask because the answer would have been terrifying.

But Colin asked and … my grief rushed out of me. Grief for my leg, grief for myself, grief for that magical thinking I'd had that maybe someday I would find a way to walk again. Grief for Emma.

'Just get yourself back into the world, Em,' he told me straight. 'You don't feel like it? Do it anyway.'

I shook my head, but I knew Colin was right.

The Lord Mayor's Ball was happening in a few weeks in aid of Debra Ireland. I was still actively the Patient Ambassador and, before the operation had even been discussed, I had bought a gorgeous olive-green jumpsuit to wear to it.

George took it out of the press and we looked at it.

'It's beautiful,' George said, hanging it up where I could see it.

I could see she was half holding her breath.

'I'm going to go,' I told her, 'I can slip in and out.'

'You could sit in the back,' she said, playing it cool.

I shouldn't have gone.

I did manage to slip in with Mom and George. We sat right at the back.

'We can leave anytime,' Mom said. My rock.

I could see Clyde and Abigail a few tables away. They turned and waved at us at one point, and I suddenly realised they might not know what had happened. I'd kept my surgery very quiet.

'I'll have to talk to Clyde,' I said.

My legs were under the table, hidden, and I felt okay, but then, suddenly, as I was chatting away to the people around me, on the big screen at the top of the room a video popped up.

The MC, Anton Savage, announced, 'One of the beneficiaries of tonight, a girl I know well and admire greatly, Emma Fogarty!'

I felt my insides drop and all I could think was, *No. Please no*. On the huge screen was a video of *me*. George leaned over and took my hand. This was nothing new, this kind of video was normal with a charity, showing the real faces behind the cause. I was used to them, I'd seen them many times, clips from years of interviews and events, cut together seamlessly into a montage with music. But where I had loved them before, now I felt like the video was mocking me. I fell apart, I kept my head down as tears dropped into my lap.

The last line of the montage was me, looking at the camera and saying, 'I just want to live.' They replayed it, that line: 'I just want to live.'

When I finally looked at Mom, she was looking at me and had tears streaming down her face. I held her arm. It was all I could do.

'I need to talk to Clyde,' I said to George, 'he doesn't know.'

I kept saying it, but I had no idea where he was.

'Let's just go,' Mom said.

As we headed out the door, Clyde was in front of me with Abigail.

He looked down and saw me in my wheelchair with my amputated leg, still recovering from surgery, lifted out in front of me.

All Clyde said over and over was, 'I didn't know, I didn't know.'

It was a huge blow to see my past life playing on the screen that night. It felt, to me, Mom and George anyway, almost like a funeral for *her*. For Emma. The one with the smile on her face. It felt like she could never come back. Losing my leg had shut a door on my old self, and she wasn't knocking to come through. Wherever she went, in some ways, she has stayed.

But you know what they say – when you hit rock bottom the only way is up. And like that phoenix you hear about in stories, I *would* rise again.

Sort of.

29

Shake it Off

Coming up to my thirty-sixth birthday I was still in despair a lot of the time, lying in bed. The pandemic wasn't helping.

'Come on, we'll go out for a walk,' George would say, and she would pull open the curtains.

'Not today,' became my motto in those dark times. I was healthy, but I wasn't my old self. I was in mourning.

But ... I was starting to stir, of course I was, and there was a new feeling in my heart that I could rebuild from this. I just had to find 'Emma' in this new version of our body. I had to lay the foundations of this new life so she could reappear.

But how?

Fundraising.

With Debra, both as a child and an adult, and as a volunteer and then Patient Ambassador, I had always been involved in fundraising. But I was never the one doing the challenges. So I decided to do something to raise money.

Myself and the team in Debra put our heads together and came up with an idea. They had a new event team, headed up by Michelle. We hadn't met in person yet.

'I was thinking I could walk a kilometre per year of my life,' I said, 'for the thirty-six days.'

She paused. Then she asked me, very casually, 'Um … but Emma … can you walk?'

I was so surprised by that question. I wanted to scream, 'Have you not spoken to the rest of Ireland? Do you not know what's happened to me?'

She *did* know, of course. She was just confused because I was suggesting something physical. I was using the word walk in a symbolic way. Michelle and I didn't know each other very well, and she hadn't learned yet how people like me talk, how we use language even when it's not completely accurate.

So I explained to her, 'No, Michelle, obviously I can't, but I could do it in my wheelchair. I could do thirty-six kilometres – one for every year I've survived.'

Daddy wasn't too sure. 'That kind of distance … the roads aren't great around here, you will hurt yourself, Emma.'

'Dad,' I said, '*that* is the challenge.'

And that was the beginning of 'Emma's 36 Challenge'.

I messaged my little group – Kim, Caitriona and Lynn.

I wrote, 'What if I raise €10 for every kilometre?'

They wrote, 'Em that's only €360!'

'No, go bigger.'

'Make it €3600.'

'That's a proper challenge.'

So we set up the *iDonate* page, set a target of €3,600 (which seemed like a crazy goal to me) and that was it. We launched the challenge in the first week of June. George pushed me on Tuesdays and Thursdays, and Mom and Dad took turns on the weekends. We figured out how to spread the thirty-six kilometres over the month, doing three or four every second or third day.

The very first week nearly killed us. The sun was splitting the stones. After one stretch, George and I were wrecked, sunburnt, totally wiped out. But we kept going and we started talking about it.

I told Ray D'Arcy, and he brought me on the radio and asked me live on air, 'What's your target?'

'€3,600,' I said.

He said, 'Let's change that to €36,000.'

I nearly fell over because he said it live. It was a target I never imagined I would hit. But I did, within the week.

Mom, Catherine and I would all sit there refreshing the page, watching the donations flood in. It climbed to €23,000 within days. Then Trisha Lewis from *Trisha's Transformation* shared it and the numbers went up again. I ended up on *The Elaine Show* too, and people just kept giving.

We wore blue every time we went out for the walk – blue hats, blue tops, anything blue – and people started calling us 'the girls in blue'.

One day in Portlaoise, four different people came up to us just to hand us a fiver or a tenner, saying, 'This is for you, girls in blue.'

It was lovely.

I got support and love from all sorts of people. I asked Colin Farrell and Johnny Sexton to make videos backing the fundraiser, and they did – that was amazing and magical in itself. I asked them to do the challenge as well.

Ray D'Arcy came back into the picture too. He wanted to do a live interview with me during one of the walks.

Of course, that day, it lashed – proper, soaking rain. I had an umbrella, but the bandages were getting wet and we couldn't risk it. We had to stop. We'd barely done two kilometres, but at least we got the interview done.

Coming up to my birthday on 25 June we realised we were nearly there, almost finished the thirty-six kilometres.

'Let's do the last four on your birthday,' Georgina said. 'No rain at all forecast, we will be grand.'

I should have known something was up. When I got up, I went into the kitchen and Catherine was sitting there with a full face of make-up on.

'Where are you going?' I asked her.

'Nowhere,' she said, innocently. So, I commented on the make-up.

'I was just trying something,' she said.

Then the doorbell went and it was my cousin Joe, all the way up from Limerick. Joe had always been a champion for me. I remember at his wedding feeling so touched to see cards on every table with the donation going to Debra Ireland.

'I was just passing,' he said this day through the door, 'I want to keep my distance.'

Joe never dropped in like that. And it was during the pandemic as well. Weird, I thought, but I was delighted to see him.

'Thanks, Joe,' I said, 'it's my birthday today!'

'What you're doing is amazing,' he said. 'I just wanted to tell you that Emma. And, of course, happy birthday.'

I was so touched to hear that from Joe. Touched that he had popped in on his way somewhere just to cheer me on, although I felt there was something, let's just say, suspect. But I ignored it, because I was so excited to finish the challenge. Joe and I took a photo together that day, standing six feet apart in the conservatory. Then he left, and myself and George went out for the last few kilometres of our challenge.

'That was so lovely to see Joe,' I said as we were parking at the hotel in town – Abbeyleix Manor – ready to take the road up around for the last few kilometres of our challenge, 'such a nice surprise.'

When we got out of the car, I saw some more people I knew, random people. My friend Pauline was there and she waved. Then I saw a group of four Debra supporters I know who call themselves 'three men and a dog' – I know them because they do the Kerry Challenge every year. They are part of the OG's, the gang who have been there from the start.

'I wonder what they're doing here?' George said as we set off. My challenge had gone viral and I thought, *Sure, maybe they just came to walk with us*. But they didn't join us, not even when I waved.

So off we went. We had four kilometres left. Two out, two back.

The walk was a good one, non-eventful. We chatted away as we went.

'Two kilometres to go to thirty-six, Emma,' George said, and I could feel her putting in extra effort.

'I can't believe we did it,' I said, 'can you, George?'

She didn't answer, because as we came around the bend we both saw a garda car covered in balloons in the road ahead. A garda got out.

'We're going to escort you,' he said.

Hmmm.

The garda car led the way, crawling along at our pace. It was surreal. At the halfway back point, another one joined us.

'What is going on?' I said.

We turned the corner then and I saw them. My whole town. Mom and Catherine had been secretly organising this surprise. There was a banner up saying, 'Well done Emma'. They'd rallied the whole town and everyone showed up, all standing six feet apart. As soon as we came into view a huge cheer erupted and my heart filled instantly, like a balloon full of their love.

Myself and George practically floated back on top of all of those cheers and well wishes.

'Come on, Emma!' I saw my school friends.

'Good on you, Emma,' I saw Orla.

'Well done, Emma!' My aunts, my cousins, my friends, neighbours, colleagues and patrons of Debra. *Wow*.

The gardaí stopped the traffic, leading and following us down the main street. People cheered the whole way, clapping, shouting 'Happy Birthday' and 'Congratulations' and 'Well done, well done, Emma!'

When we got back to that hotel where we'd parked earlier, there was another crowd waiting for us. Including the three men and a dog.

'I knew it was weird to see ye here,' I said as I passed them.

I saw Joe.

'I knew it was weird to see you too!' I waved at him.

The whole town was packed. Bunting, balloons, signs saying, 'Well done Emma'. Mom and Catherine had formed a whole committee to pull it off.

I remember turning to George, overwhelmed in the best way, saying, 'How did I not see this coming?'

Of course, I hadn't prepared a speech, but I went up in front of everyone and did my best. At one point, a nervous young garda stood beside me.

'I'm so glad to see people up from Dublin and Limerick,' I said, looking at the garda, and then said, 'I probably shouldn't have said that.'

Everyone burst out laughing, totally breaking the tension that was everywhere in the early days of the pandemic.

We had a small party afterwards at the house. Pandemic restrictions meant we had to keep it outside and limit the numbers, but it didn't matter. That day was enough.

The same day, Colin ran thirty-six kilometres on the treadmill. As for Johnny, well, I'm still waiting!

We finished having raised €106,000. From €3,600 to €106,000. 'Emma's 36 Challenge' was done. In more ways than one.

And *I* was starting again, finally.

29

Sky Full of Stars

I love music so much. I couldn't live without it. I know everyone says that, but I mean it – when I put on music, I am anywhere and anyone. I'm on stage with a crowd in front of me. I'm in a film. I'm on a beach running into the waves. I'm under the stars around a bonfire with my friends. I'm in love.

It's magical. A lifesaver.

If I'm in agony, and that's often, I don't turn on the TV. My family know this: if it's quiet in my room I have my headphones on.

As you know, Mom used to sing to me in bed when I was little and suffering, trying to sleep. Her voice was so soothing. And whenever we were in the car my parents would play a tape of children's songs and we would all sing along. Once it ran through both sides I would shout, 'Again!', and my dad would turn it over and start the songs playing all over again, until eventually they'd get tired of that and put on their own music. As I got older, we all played whatever we wanted.

My memories are shaped by music – my solace, my escape. It takes me away to another place, outside of this body. It lets me relax. It lets me pretend. Music creates a bubble between my soul and my pain and holds us at a distance for a while.

I always shuffle music. I don't mind what it is, surprise me

Apple Music, I love nearly all of it. The only thing I don't like is opera and heavy rock, but I'll listen to almost anything else.

My first concert was Justin Timberlake. I went with my support worker, Dominique, and we had so much fun. I could still walk at that point and we spent the whole concert dancing. From then on, I was fully hooked on concerts. Concerts are really accessible in Ireland, which means the world to me. There is always an area for wheelchairs where I can go and feel safe. The only problem is it's always too far away, never in the thick of it.

I've seen Taylor Swift, Pink, Adele, Westlife, Michael Bublé, so many. I was supposed to go to Beyoncé for a third time with Lynn. That's the only concert EB stopped me from making. I was too ill in hospital to go and I was raging. I hate those moments when EB shows me who is boss.

When Pink came to Dublin I was dying to see her. She was playing the RDS and there wasn't a ticket to be had. I sat up for them like most people but ... oh my God that queue! I couldn't get tickets, so, with fighting spirit, I put the word out on Twitter, hoping for a miracle.

Then a neighbour from Abbeyleix reached out with tickets. I could not believe my luck. She was so kind and refused to take any money from us, even though we almost had an argument over that!

When we got to Dublin on the day of the concert, our neighbour was waiting for us and brought us – me, Mom, Georgina and Pauline – right to our seats.

We thought we'd be in the usual wheelchair section, but instead she led us into this gorgeous VIP area. It was really lush, and waiters kept bringing out canapés and food – every time we ate or drank something, more arrived. Wine. More wine. Even more wine. Anything you wanted to eat and drink, you could get.

The gig hadn't even started yet, and we were already having the time of our lives.

When Pink came on … wow. The energy she has to sing, to dance, she even flew around our heads on a rope, it was wild. We were a bit disappointed she didn't talk to us more – I think she only said, 'Hello, Dublin' – but watching her was incredible all the same. She did all the hits, and we were up dancing, singing, taking photos, laughing.

Mom was in her element; she loves Pink and always has. We all do, but Mom was especially giddy that night because of the swish section from which we were watching the concert. She was belting out the tracks, waving every time Pink swung by us.

'How much wine has Mom had?' I said with a giggle.

We had all had more than one glass and it livened us up for sure. I was singing along too, able to stand for a few songs even, it was one of those nights where the energy just carries you.

At one point I heard someone calling my name. We were up high in a kind of square viewing area above the crowd. I looked down and there was Sarah, my good friend and a supporter of Debra. She was waving up at me, shouting, 'Emma! Emma!'

Sarah is one of those people who, when I met her, I instantly loved her. I was delighted to see her at Pink.

'I'm coming up!' she called and then disappeared. About ten minutes later, she burst in, breathless. 'I've gone through about ten doors trying to find you!' We all knew her, so there were hugs all round.

'I saw your yellow blouse,' she said, 'and I was like, that's my Emma!' She stayed to watch the concert with us.

Mom was still having the time of her life – and maybe enjoying the wine a little more than usual. George was driving us halfway home, dropping us to my car, but it became very clear very fast that Mom, who was supposed to drive the rest of the way, would *not* be driving anywhere that night. She was dancing and waving and getting closer and closer to this little gap at the edge of the platform. I kept trying to pull her back, but she was three sheets to the wind by then, impossible to manage.

'We need coffee. Quick,' Georgina said.

Outside the VIP section we could see a coffee stall, and so Sarah lifted herself up to jump over the fence – and Mom, not to be outdone, decided she could do it too. She threw her leg over, lost her balance and landed on top of *me*, flat across my lap, looking up at me. She started howling with laughter. Absolutely howling.

'I don't want coffee,' she kept saying, waving us off. None of us could stop laughing. We forced a cup of coffee into her.

Later, we made it back to the car. I needed to take my medication, but we had no water to flush the syringe. Without missing a beat, Mom searched around my car, grabbed a bottle of prosecco that I happened to have in the back seat, and flushed the syringe with that.

I was laughing so hard I nearly passed out. I kept thinking, *WHO is this woman and where is my mother?* Needless to say, Mom remembers *none* of this.

George had to drive us all the way back to Abbeyleix in my car, with Mom insisting from the back seat that she was perfectly fine. Then George had to head back to the hotel car park to leave my car and collect her own.

'I'll collect it in the morning,' Mom swore.

But the next morning, she messaged, 'Can you bring Emma's car? I'm too tired to drive.'

So, 'tired' is what we're calling it nowadays ...

Those memories are some of my favourites, just the absolute chaos and fun we had. I love moments when things are real, not careful, not deliberate or cautious. I love mayhem because it brings me inside the fold where all of you are, instead of being on the outside.

Pink really puts on a show. I'm so grateful to her for the effort she puts in – it's not just the performance; it's the whole experience.

* * *

Mom loves Coldplay. She has always loved hearing them on the radio, and so, when they came to Dublin in 2024, I thought, *I'll do anything to get her there.*

Things were tough for me at the time, EB wise, emotion wise, but I didn't care, I really wanted to go with Mom regardless. So I hunted around, I even put a call out on Twitter (Mom's not on there) and, eventually, a patron of Debra Ireland who I know really well, a guardian angel (I won't say who because he would kill me) got me tickets.

I teased Mom a bit before I told her.

'If you had to play golf,' I asked her as we sat in the kitchen, 'where would you go?'

She laughed. 'What? Golf?'

'Yeah, if you could go anywhere to play, where would you go?'

'Florida,' she said.

'Okay,' I said. 'Then what is your dream holiday?'

'Florida.' She played along.

'Okay,' I said, 'if you could go to any restaurant?'

'Em ...' she had to think about that one. 'Harts,' she said.

'What concert would you go to?'

'Coldplay,' she said, 'in a heartbeat.'

'But that's next week,' I replied. 'Tickets are sold out.'

'Ah well,' she said.

I kept the questions going.

'If you'd to go on a cruise,' I said, 'where would you go?'

She winked, 'Florida.'

'If you ...' I was running out of questions, 'could go to any holiday place?'

'You asked me that,' she said, suspicious now. 'What's this about?'

'One of your answers is going to happen,' I said. 'Think of what you said – and didn't say.'

She couldn't remember and to be honest neither could I, except one.

So I just told her. 'We're going to Coldplay.'

Her face dropped. She had to hold on to the back of the chair.

'Are you kidding me?' she said.

'No,' I said, 'I'm not. We are going.'

Her face lit up like a child at Christmas getting the present she always wanted.

'Are you *kidding* me?' She could not believe it.

I was in a lot of pain the day of the concert, but we still had a ball. Mom loved it. There were balloons floating around the crowd, giant inflatable balls we batted around. We laughed and danced and forgot about EB for a while. She knew all the songs, except the new ones. Aslan came out as special guests. It was two-for-one.

'They're the best band I've ever seen,' she said.

Mom has given up so much for me. That night was something I could give her. I will never be able to thank my guardian-*Bobby-Healy*-shaped angel enough for getting me the tickets. (Sorry, Bobby, but I couldn't not put you in here!)

I am just so happy that I live in a country where singers can come to perform. It is so wonderful that they put in all this effort to entertain us. And I am grateful to venues in Ireland that are so accessible, which means people with restrictions can enjoy them safely, just like everyone else.

I don't take that for granted. Not for a second.

***

One of the best concerts I ever went to was Ed Sheeran. One man and a guitar, filling the stage with total presence. His album *Divide* is actually one of my favourites of all time, as in it's in my top three. Ed's part-Irish. I love that and I think it makes that connection you don't get with others.

I remember seeing that he had done a concert in aid of EB for his friend Courteney Cox. Someone really close to Courteney had a child with EB and Ed had played for a fundraiser. It endeared him to me for sure, but then when *Equals* came out, something just clicked. It felt like a spark – like his masterpiece. I thought, *This is it. I'm going to meet him.* I just knew. The butterfly on the album cover? I took it as a sign. The idea of meeting him got into my head and I was so motivated. I can't describe it, it was this will, and I'm never pushy but I really decided to put pressure on everyone, including Jimmy, to make it happen. Jimmy really tried. We all did.

The night before his concert, I texted Jimmy, 'I don't think it's going to happen. I'm giving up.'

I couldn't believe it. I had been so convinced that I would meet my hero. It had felt so obvious to me, of course I would. But now I was starting to accept that it was way too much to ask of the universe.

About half an hour later, I got a message from someone else: 'I might have some information. Give me a minute.'

Then another message: 'I know where he's having lunch.' She said where it was.

I couldn't believe it, Osteria Lucio. That place was only five doors down from Debra's office. I was shaking.

I FaceTimed George.

'George,' I said, 'can we change our plans for tomorrow? Can you bring me to Dublin to meet Ed Sheeran, please? Pretty please?'

'Of course,' she said.

The next morning in Dublin, George parked in the Debra wheelchair spot. Then George and I, along with Mom, who had decided to come too, sat in the car wondering how to best approach this ambush.

I was terrified Ed was already in there. I kept thinking he would suddenly come out and go, and we'd miss him because I couldn't get out of the car fast enough.

'I'll block him in if that happens,' George said.

Just then a black van pulled up. Ed Sheeran jumped out and ran inside the restaurant.

'Oh myyyy GODDDD!' I shrieked.

'That's the man we want,' George said. 'Right.'

She turned off the car, got out and got me out, into my wheelchair and onto the footpath.

'I can't believe he is in there,' I just kept repeating that.

Then a woman approached, the one who had texted. We all felt like spies at this stage – I swear it is funny in the retelling, but at the time you'd think we had the outcome of the Cold War on our shoulders.

'Drive behind the van,' she said out of the corner of her mouth, 'and just have Emma on the path there by the door, sitting talking.'

'It's a free country,' George said, getting the gist of the plan. She wheeled me over while Mom turned the car and parked. There we were. We tried not to be too obvious, keeping one eye on the restaurant door. I sat talking to Mom through the window of the car, as if I had just been going that way and spotted an old friend, but as time passed it got harder to make it look natural.

The driver of the black van kept looking at us over his shoulder. I widened my eyes at George and she held on to the handles of my chair.

'And how is Malachy?' she said to my mom, buying us a few more minutes. Next thing, the van driver approached us, but he stopped just before he got to us. Then he spoke out of the corner of his mouth.

'Open your back window,' he hissed to Mom. She did, and he quickly headed back to the van, then returned with an armful of merch, which he threw in the window. It was all so quick.

'You don't know where those came from,' he said over his shoulder as he went back to the van.

I was on a high. Everyone was on our side, this was going to happen.

Suddenly, Ed was on the street. He looked over and waved.

'Hi guys,' he said, and he didn't just leave like he could have, like he was planning to do before he saw us. Instead, he stopped and came over. 'Want anything signed?'

'Hi, I'm Emma,' I introduced myself, 'and this is my mom and this is Georgina.'

Ed signed a poster and took selfies with us, including one on his own phone.

I remember grabbing his sleeve to hold him. I suddenly decided I wanted to talk about his connection to EB.

'You did a concert for EB,' I said, 'thank you for spreading awareness.'

'That's a pleasure,' he said, 'it's a great cause, I was happy to.'

'I'm going to your show tonight,' I said.

'I hope you enjoy it,' he said and turned to go. But I held onto his arm. I decided to be brazen.

'I might ask you to do another someday – for Debra.'

He laughed. 'Definitely,' he said.

I wanted to set a date right there and then, but I bottled out of pushing him any more. I let go of his sleeve and, with a big wave, Ed Sheeran left in the van.

I wish I'd had more time to talk to him. I would love the chance to tell him how much his music means to me – especially the song 'Visiting Hours'. So many of his songs feel like they were written for me. They're bops sure – I can't believe I just used that word – but they're also genius. His lyrics are incredible, and they really get inside my soul. I believe every word and I feel every word. His concert that night was amazing, although it was so cold, and we loved every minute.

When he's back, I'll be there. If he'd just give me 30 minutes, I have an idea for a fundraiser I'd give anything to pitch to him. And like I do with most people in the limelight, I'd tell him all about EB. But I would also tell him just how much his music helped me survive.

Thank you, Ed.

30

Visiting Hours

EB chips away at things over time. Your movement, your quality of living, your self-esteem, your mental health. It comes to get you, one freedom at a time.

And then you start again, like a castaway from some terrible shipwreck, and build a new life around what you have left.

That's what I've done. What I'm still doing. I live in hope and wait for EB when it decides to take something else. It is always the boss of me.

As EB patients live out our lives and get older, things can become more complicated, especially for people like me with the more severe forms. Wounds that once healed, even if slowly, might now stay open for longer, or never fully close at all. And, of course, chronic wounds can become infected easily, and managing them is a never-ending, daily, time-consuming routine. Scarring builds up over time, often pulling the skin tighter and limiting movement. We get things called contractures – where the skin and muscles tighten so much that our movement is really limited.

It's not just the skin on the outside that's affected either – the linings inside the body can become more fragile too (if that is possible), so things like eating, swallowing, those hardships that plague us from childhood, become impossible.

Some people with EB deal with much worse internal issues than I have had. I've been so lucky that way, they have it much harder because there are no bandages for the inside, you can't support your organs by wrapping them.

We always have to keep an eye out for wounds that won't heal. Getting cancer, as I knew full well, can prove fatal. Still, I find checking to be just as traumatic – since Bobby passed away, since my first cancer diagnosis, since losing my leg – I try to avoid investigation. I've asked myself whether it's because I want to avoid the feeling of dread when you hear that word. Is it that I think if I don't know it isn't real? I'm not sure.

Or maybe I just can't face more poking and prodding. Maybe my amygdala is working in overdrive.

I know that I resist investigation because I just want to live. It's counter-productive, I know. It makes no sense, but hopefully there is a part of you that will get it. I am human. I avoid what scares me.

After going to Lourdes at eighteen, I had barely choked at all. Isn't that amazing? For almost twenty years I could eat almost anything I liked, even if that was still mostly soft things. I wasn't eating steak or nachos, I never had the nerve. But I'd happily munch away on chocolate or soft crisps, and of course my beloved chicken wings and soft fried potatoes. It was great and made me part of the world again in a way I had missed so much.

Then, at thirty-eight, I suddenly found myself back there, in a world where I could barely manage soup. I couldn't even sip a little 7UP. (Can I just say, I should be sponsored by 7UP, I drink so much of it.) I would take a little mouthful and choke. It was hell. What was happening?

At first I waited for it to pass, but eventually I admitted defeat and rang Professor Ravi, my gastroenterologist.

He was surprised.

'I can still drink coffee,' I told him, willing him to reassure me.

'I don't like the sound of any of this, Emma,' he admitted, 'and yes, maybe it is a temperature thing ... if you want to wait and see, I'm happy for you to do that.'

He knew not to push.

We kept in touch over the summer and into the autumn, with him calling every few weeks to ask me how I was. By October things were not improving at all. In fact, they were getting worse. You could tell, because instead of waiting for him to ask, I told him how I was. I admitted defeat.

'I'm not great,' I said, 'I'm not really able to drink now.'

'Emma,' he said, and I heard his tone sharpen to real concern, 'if you can't manage a drink I need to see you. This could be the point of no return, we need to get you in here as soon as possible.'

That phrase – the point of no return – hit me like a thump in the chest.

'Okay,' I started to panic, 'please get me in soon.'

They did.

* * *

Usually, I get knocked out for any sort of investigations with a cannula into my vein, both for my benefit and theirs. My childhood fear of the surgical mask is genuine. It's not easy for doctors to deal with a patient who is panicking and, no matter how much I prepare myself, I go mental whenever a mask is put on my face.

I'm kind to myself on that level. I have been through an awful lot, both as a child and as an adult, and I'm only human at the end of the day, so when they ask, I just say, 'No.' It has never been a problem. Normally, they inject sedatives directly into my vein and knock me out that way.

This time, however, they couldn't find one. Of course they couldn't! I had been fasting, with no food or water, since the night before. My veins were nowhere to be seen.

The anaesthetist said, 'Emma, would you let us *try* a mask?'

My inner child said, 'No.'

After a few further attempts to find a vein, they went and got my mother, who came in and, bless her, tried to coax me.

'Just try it once,' she suggested.

No go.

'I don't want to,' I said. 'No.'

I was even trying to coax myself in my head, talking to myself as an adult thinking, *Just do it*, but my inner child was having none of it.

'No,' she said.

'How about if I hold it just here?' the doctor said, trying a trick. He waved it around about a foot above me. I know masks don't hurt, but my terror is real. Phobias aren't rational, they're visceral. One smell of that gas and my childhood instincts flood back. I started to cry.

'No,' I said, 'please.'

My mom tried it on herself. 'It's fine, Emma, see? Please just try.'

'No,' I said, 'please, I don't want to wear it.'

'It doesn't hurt, Emma,' the anaesthetist said, and I saw him looking at the clock, 'just please let me hold it up here.'

He held it up above my head.

I held my breath and let him wave it around a foot away. Then he turned on the gas.

'No,' I said, feeling the flow on my face, 'please.'

I thought the man had lost his mind then, because he started this random conversation with me, asking me loads of questions about myself, such as where I was living. I remember at the time thinking, *What are you on, pal?*

Now, of course, I know what he was doing. When you speak, you breathe, and, being as flustered as I was, each answer I gave him was followed by a large inhale of breath … and gas.

'Abbeyleix.' Inhale.

'Just me and my sister.' Inhale.

'Business.' Inhale again, and I felt Mom patting my arm.

'Thirty … eighttttsssshhh …' I was starting to slur.

The mask was brought down to about ten inches.

'Just a bit of gas, just get yourself drowsy,' he said.

Mom held my hand.

'Mom,' I said, 'I don't want to …'

But my eyes were closing.

I told her I loved her. I said. 'Goodbye, Mom.'

And then … gone. I don't remember anything after that, but they told me I kept talking while I was under.

I woke in recovery, vomiting blood. Nurses kept pulling my hair.

'Stop,' I told them.

Professor Ravi came to see me.

'Emma,' he said, and his face was so serious it frightened me, 'the throat of most adults is the size of a grape, four centimetres.'

I knew what was coming.

'Your throat was four millimetres. We caught this just in time.'

Thank God they investigated when they did. Four millimetres

is unliveable. If it had closed any further I would have spent the rest of my life unable to eat or drink.

Every few hours nurses would come in and fuss around me. I wasn't exactly bouncing back, let's just put it that way. My throat was on fire, my stomach was in terrible pain from all the blood it had swallowed, and the nurses *kept* pulling my hair.

'Mom,' I called out at one point, 'tell them to stop pulling my hair.'

'Emma, pet,' she leaned down, 'the only vein they could find was in your head.'

I had no idea I even had veins in my head, but there you go. I freaked out a little when she told me that, but they had to give me the meds somehow.

Of course, regardless of needing sleep and recovery, I was still on call for EB. I had to do a bandage change that same morning, taking breaks to vomit blood into a bowl. George and my mom did it, because the only EB nurse in St James's Hospital was on holiday.

Thankfully, after the bandage change I was allowed home.

Now I can't eat at all. I have a little soft white chocolate sometimes, or a few Dairy Milk Buttons to melt in my mouth.

And if I am at a meal, I will see if they have soup and if they do I will ask them to strain it through a sieve. It drives me cracked because so many times when I ask them, they'll reply straight away with, 'Oh, it's already blended.'

And I say, 'Can you please just strain it anyway?'

I hate having to beg and I hate having to explain why I am asking.

31

Breathe

In July 2023 I woke up one morning, just after my thirty-ninth birthday, to read that Taylor Swift had announced Dublin dates for the week of my fortieth birthday. The whole of Ireland was out to get some, and so Ticketmaster had arranged a system of codes. I applied, I waited. I didn't get one. Like half the country, I was really disappointed. Taylor meant so much to me.

Then, my nurses arrived to do bandages and one of them, Simone, said, 'Did you get the code?'

I told her about my disappointment. 'Did you get it?'

'I did,' she said. 'It lets you buy four, but I'm only getting two, so you can have the other two.'

I nearly fell out of my bed, I'm telling you. I couldn't believe it. We were meant to be starting bandages, but instead we were straight on to Ticketmaster, trying to sort it. The other nurse was like, 'Hellooooo …'

I could not believe I was this lucky. I was going to see Taylor. I was one of the chosen few. It felt like I was going to see God or something – dramatic I know, but just so magical.

'I'll bring Catherine,' I said. It was perfect.

Just after we got the tickets – feeling like I was on cloud nine – I woke up one morning struggling to breathe. I did not know what was wrong with me. It felt like a heavy cold, or a flu.

One of the nurses at the time who would come to help with my bandages was a strange character, it was almost as if she thought that I was putting on my suffering. I mean, come on, look at me!

It always felt to me like she didn't believe me if I told her I wasn't great or that I was in extra pain when she asked. And that attitude meant that I stopped complaining. Which is such a dangerous thing. Imagine not feeling free to tell a nurse how you are really feeling.

This one Monday morning I did complain. Because I could hardly breathe.

'I'm not feeling great,' I said.

'You're grand,' she said, not even really looking at me.

'I can't breathe,' I said.

'You're grand,' she said again.

As she changed my bandages, I put my hand on my chest and through my ribs I could feel my heart pounding. It felt like it was trying to drill through my ribs, it was pounding that hard.

'I think my heart is pounding,' I said.

This nurse met the eyes of the other one who was helping that day. 'This one is always looking for problems,' she said.

When she was done with the bandage change, she left.

'Emma,' my mom felt my forehead, 'will I call the doctor?'

'No,' I said, really not wanting another stint in hospital, 'I'll probably be grand tomorrow.'

That nurse's reluctance had given me this idea that I must be overreacting. A nurse would never ignore a real issue, would she?

Mom knows there is no point in pushing me. So she just

kept an eye on me the whole day, popping her head in and checking every few minutes that I was alright. I played it cool. 'I'm fine. Much better.'

But by the time George came in on Tuesday morning I couldn't get through a sentence without becoming so breathless I felt dizzy.

George took one look at me and I could tell she wasn't happy. 'Emma, are you okay?' she said.

I'd been suffering for two days and really didn't feel well, so I agreed to call the doctor. At that time I was the only adult with EB in the country. All the other sufferers were under twenty and still going to the paediatric hospital, so I was under the care of a team that wasn't focused on EB, unlike the team in Crumlin. The hospitals in Dublin wouldn't be ready for me and they wouldn't understand EB, and this, many times, has led to real suffering for me. So I always try to avoid hospital.

But I called Mr Ormonde.

'If I said I wanted you to come in, would you?' he said. He knows me well.

'Yes,' I said.

'Okay, well,' he said, 'I want you to come straight away.'

'Okay,' I said.

As Georgina was helping me get ready to go, she put her hands on my back and I heard her gasp.

'Emma,' she said, and her voice sounded really serious, 'your heart feels like a bird trying to get out a window, I swear.'

'I told … the … nurse,' I said. Each word was a real struggle by that stage.

Mom and Dad got me into the car and we went straight up to St James's Hospital.

When we arrived, Mr Ormonde had called down and they

were waiting for me. They had an airbed and everything set up and luckily there was a room too.

'I'd say you'll be home tomorrow,' he said, 'it could be a chest infection.'

On went the ECG machine and I saw Mom's face fall when the numbers hit the screen. I had a resting pulse of 155. Double the norm.

So the tests started. They did an X-ray with a machine they brought into the room, which was brilliant because I was exhausted. I was tested for everything, including Covid.

'You have pneumonia,' Mr Ormonde said, 'you'll have to stay in as we need to treat it with strong antibiotics.'

After he left, a team from the ICU came in and that really scared me. The nurse assured me, 'We're just checking in to see how you are.'

I'd never seen the ICU. I knew something wasn't right. The pain I was feeling wasn't normal. I know what EB feels like and, of course, I take strong drugs to dull it. But even so, I could sense something else, like a crawling sensation through me.

What was wrong with me?

Halfway through the day I started begging for pain medication, but they just wouldn't bring any. It had been hours since I'd missed my normal dose. Mom had brought enough for the morning, thinking I would be fine in a hospital. I mean you'd think so right? You'd presume the hospital could give me a replacement. Silly me.

On and on, the pain mounted, but every time I asked for something, they acted like I was acting or not being sincere, and they refused to give me any relief.

'You've had a paracetamol,' one nurse said looking at the chart.

'I need my medication,' I explained.

'We don't have that sort of medication in A&E,' the nurse said.

'I have EB,' I said, 'I take it five times a day, I just didn't bring it because I thought I would be going home.'

She just gave me this look and left the room. Left for the first time in years without any pain relief, I was bawling.

Where was Colin Farrell and that 'look' when I needed him?

You know, I get it, the nurse had no idea that pain from EB at my stage feels like you are actually being flayed alive. She didn't know that at my stage, EB patients *need* strong pain relief just to sit calmly. We don't suffer only one kind of pain – we suffer layers of pain happening all at once. Blisters and open wounds feel like burns. The skin can sting, throb or feel raw, like it's been badly scraped or scalded. Even a small touch or a shift in clothing can feel like fire. Sometimes skin tears just from being moved or touched – like if you accidentally pull off a plaster, except it's your actual skin. That ripping pain can be sharp and shocking. Open wounds that never fully heal are always sore. They itch and hurt all the time, dull but constant. As if that wasn't enough, there is also nerve involvement around scar tissue. It's like cold white heat, electric-shock sensations, or pain that shoots through my body without warning.

You know these types of pain – hot nerve endings, exposed wounds, that heavy presence under a plaster when you've cut yourself. In severe forms of EB, like mine, swallowing can feel like swallowing glass. Going to the loo can be agony. Even breathing deeply hurts when the lining of my nose is affected.

I don't think nurses who don't know what they're dealing

with should be allowed to say no to patients. There should be a hotline they can call, at least, to make sure these kinds of situations can be managed.

Eventually – I think just to shut me up – the nurse relented. She gave me one dose of strong pain relief. I usually get the equivalent of five doses – when it wears off the pain is actually indescribable. But it was something. However, it wore off really quickly and the nurse I had convinced earlier had finished her shift and now I had to convince a new one all over again. It all felt so cruel.

Thankfully, they moved me up to the ward I know well: Haematology & Hepatology. We call it 'The H & H'. It's a specialised ward for patients with blood-clotting disorders. But as I was the only adult EB patient in Ireland, I always went in there. I knew the nurses, they knew me.

A few moments after I arrived a nurse popped her head in.

'Do you need anything, Emma?' she said.

'Can I have my medication?' I begged. My voice broke with the stress of waiting.

'Of course,' she said and went off, returning with a full dose in moments. I was so relieved.

'I love you,' I said.

***

The next day Mr Ormonde came in and I knew by his face that something was not good. I braced myself.

'Emma,' he said, 'we have found sepsis in your bloodstream …'

My whole body reacted to those words; I barely heard the rest of the sentence.

'… but we are on top of it …'

I know a lot about sepsis. Probably too much to hear it so casually.

'… and we caught it early.'

I was so scared to hear that.

Mr Ormonde told me, 'It would have spread quickly.'

I remember feeling really lucky. If I hadn't had pneumonia and not been able to breathe, they would never have found the beginning of the sepsis.

'What made you tell me to come in?' I asked him then.

'The fact that you said you would,' he said. 'I've fought far too many battles trying to get you to come in in the past, so I knew straight away you must be bad to want to come.'

I'd never had pneumonia or sepsis before in my life, and I haven't since. I really think someone was looking after me that time.

Hopefully Bobby.

32

Begin Again

As soon as I turned thirty-nine, I started thinking about turning forty.

Forty is a massive milestone for any woman. For me it was an age I never thought I'd see. Forty is extraordinary for people with EB. I'd spent my twenties and thirties haunted by how fast Bobby was taken from us and feeling certain the same would happen to me. So, coming up to forty was not just a milestone, it was a feat. I wanted to do something to mark it, something that would lift everyone's spirits.

I planned the normal celebrations, the dinners out and drinks. I knew I wanted to celebrate with Colin. We couldn't really go for dinner, I can't eat. We couldn't go for drinks, he doesn't drink. I kept thinking about something he had said a few years earlier – how he'd love to run the Dublin marathon. Could I do the marathon too?

No. There was no way I could survive in my chair for forty-two kilometres.

'Maybe you could do a forty challenge?' Pauline suggested. 'Like the thirty-six, a few every day.'

'No,' I said, 'it has to be bigger, larger and really fun.'

I couldn't do the marathon, I knew I couldn't, but I just could not stop dreaming about it.

So, of course, I asked Colin to do it for me instead.

'Hi Col, how are you?' I asked him in a voice note. 'Any chance you'd run the marathon for my fortieth?'

I paused, 'And push me for the last four K … one K for every decade?'

He responded with his news, the bits and bobs he was up to, all the usual stuff, and then he said, 'That little question you slid into your message, I'd love to, but with the strike and I'm doing two movies … I just don't know will the timing work – when is it?'

When he heard the date he sent a text.

'Em, I will be working that whole time … I can't.'

I heard him, but it didn't feel like all was lost. I didn't feel down. It was like, inside, I knew this dream would come true.

'I would if I could, you know that,' he said.

'Look,' I replied, 'it was one idea, I will come up with something else, don't worry.'

* * *

Mom and I, George and I, Catherine and I brainstormed every chance we got. Nothing came close to my first idea.

Then, late one morning, I got a voice note from Colin.

'Emma,' he said, 'I'm in New York, lying here in bed, and I just can't stop thinking about your idea that we would do the marathon together.'

I put my volume up as high as it would go. I was also lying there thinking about my idea. I was also lying there wishing I could run the marathon with Colin.

'I've a few things on,' he told me, 'the movie, and there's something else in the pipeline with dates that clash but …' he lowered his voice, 'I have this feeling – depending on how things fall – that I could ... we might be able to do this.'

I held my breath.

'How amazing would it be,' he went on, 'if we crossed that finish line together?'

I realised there was a second voice note, just after his first one.

He had an idea.

'Why don't we go all out?' he suggested. 'If we are going to do this, let's go all out. Emma, let's make a documentary!'

I exhaled in a rush and sent a voice note back to him. 'That sounds amazing,' I said.

It had never been on my bucket list to do a documentary (unlike this book, which has been on the list for years). I hadn't ever even thought about that. But now I wanted to. It sounded like a brilliant plan.

'It's not going to be easy, Em,' Colin said.

'I know,' I said, 'but sure, what ever is?'

After that wonderful time, the countdown was on to the marathon.

'Emma, I can't push you in your normal chair,' he said, on the phone one day, 'we have to get a sports chair. An all-terrain yoke.'

I really didn't want to. Like, I really, *really* didn't.

'I don't want the sports chair,' I said, 'they look like a huge baby buggy.'

'They don't.' Colin knew what was going on. He knows me. He knows well that I feel humiliated as a disabled person.

I know it's silly, but I do. It's who I am. I have that spot in my heart that still thrives on independence, and anything that reduces me, anything that makes me feel babied, is deeply hard on my soul. I suppose I have so little adult life, so little adulthood in the way that I rely so much on other people for everything. So visual things like that – being strapped into a huge buggy – hurt me to my core. Maybe it sounds mad, but that's how it is. Take me or leave me, I am who I am.

'I can't push you in that manual chair,' Colin insisted, 'it'll hurt you too much.'

'Colin, listen,' I said, 'I could turn over in bed and tear my shoulder off, or my hip. You know this. I could bump into someone in a shop or anything. I want to do this with you.'

* * *

I turned forty in June 2024. I didn't want a big bash, I had the Taylor Swift tickets, and the marathon, in October, was going to be the climax of my life, I knew that much – so I told everyone I just wanted to keep things small.

'A few glasses of prosecco on the day,' I said.

My dear friends Perry and Sandy had other ideas. They organised a party for me in Kilkee Castle and a small group of us went down for the weekend. It was so special.

A few days later, we were filming for the marathon documentary, and I looked up and everyone was smiling. A huge bouquet of flowers was set down in the conservatory – pink, cream and green, bigger than anything I'd ever seen. It was easily a hundred euro-worth of flowers.

And at that exact moment Colin FaceTimed me and said, 'Happy birthday.'

'Oh wow,' I said, 'Colin, thank you, I love the flowers.'

He started smiling and I sensed something was up, 'Well, Emma,' he said, 'I've got you executive tickets for Taylor Swift.'

I didn't know what an executive ticket was, but I started crying because it was all so lovely and thoughtful. I wanted to bring Mom. Catherine was still coming of course – I couldn't keep her away. The documentary crew wanted to come too, to film us there, though they would have to do it on their phone since you couldn't go in with film cameras.

I gave the two tickets I already had to a little girl with the same form of EB I have, Casey. She was at that perfect age for a concert. I knew she loved Taylor. I called her mom.

'Did Casey get tickets for Taylor?' I said.

She replied with a sad no. I knew that feeling, I'd felt it myself the year before when the tickets went on sale.

'Do you want two?' I said.

I don't think I could make one word out in the answer, they were so excited. It was a blessing that I had got those tickets, and it was a blessing to pass them on to another person with EB. Colin didn't just give me the joy of Taylor Swift when he bought me such a wonderful present, he gave me the joy of being able to make dreams come true for someone else, as has happened so many times for me.

When we arrived at Croke Park I found out what an executive ticket is – Colin had bought us a whole box! We had seats in there and everything we needed, and a great view of the entire stage, which was enormous – it looked a mile long. Can you believe Colin did that for me? He is amazing.

Taylor Swift was beyond belief. I knew every song. It felt like a pure, innocent night. A big dancing moment. A free bar didn't hurt either. I really think it was the best night of my life. She played for three hours. She took zero breaks. The way the whole show was set up showed me that she really, really cares about her fans, she wants to give every performance her all and put on a real show. And she did! She even dove into the stage – I don't know how she did it – and it looked like she was swimming.

Not long after that Colin came home and we met in the Killashee. He took me for a spin on the smooth roads of the hotel grounds.

'Okay,' he said, and he started to jog, 'let's try it out.'

We went so fast. It was really fun.

'Will I let go?' Colin joked.

I said, 'Go on then.' And then I saw his two hands waving on either side of my face for just a moment. I laughed so hard I almost fell out of my wheelchair.

'How *is* the chair?' Colin said.

'Grand,' I lied. Within seconds of Colin starting to run I had really felt the difference.

'Emma, I don't know about this,' Colin said, slowing down a bit and turning. *Colin might be right*, I thought, finally understanding that I would have to give in. Being pushed when someone is running creates so much friction, even on the smoothest roads.

Colin noticed me yelp as we ran along. He stopped. Now I got that 'look' myself.

'This won't work, Emma,' he said.

A few days after that, I was crossing the road at home in my wheelchair and I really thought about it. Those few moments across that old road were fairly hard for me on a daily basis. I imagined going down it for four kilometres. Colin *was* right. I knew this challenge would either have to be as a baby in a big buggy or not at all. I knew I'd have to put up with the sports chair. I would have to swallow my pride and just do it.

I finally admitted it.

'Okay,' I said, 'I'll go in the sports chair.'

'Good woman,' Colin said.

The Irish Wheelchair Association adapted a sports wheelchair especially for me. They padded it out with soft flexible foam and put in a special piece for my little leg, all padded out too, to keep me safe. Because my left leg doesn't go straight down, they added a little cushion behind it and taped it in, so it stayed secure. Every part of that chair was shaped and angled to fit me perfectly.

I didn't feel great in it, I won't lie. But I got it, I knew why I was there, and if I looked like a baby, well I would laugh about it afterwards.

The wheelchair didn't solve one problem. This was still an extreme sport and if one step was wrong, or if someone hit off Colin and made him hit off the chair, I could fall out.

If my wheel went too close to a railing, if the chair hit the curb or if the road dipped where you couldn't see it – it didn't bear thinking about how it could end if I was tipped over at the speed of Colin running. But I didn't care. I wanted to do it anyway.

Colin, though, was feeling the pressure.

'If I spill Emma, it's curtains,' he said.

33

I Lived

The week before the marathon, Colin flew home. The documentary crew started rolling straight away. There were loads of crew. I gave them all nicknames to remember who was who. 'Mick the mic guy,' I'd say as soon as he would appear to clip on the microphone that I would wear all day. We had 'Irish Shane' and 'American Shane' doing the video. Every single thing was recorded, so we had to be careful. Mick could hear *everything*.

The activity at the house was non-stop. So many people, so much gear and cords running around, make-up bags and takeaway coffees all over.

We did one or two official things – I remember collecting a cheque from Irish Life. We took photos with the gardaí, we talked on Ray D'Arcy, we met the chief of the Dublin marathon, Jim Aughney, who was a total gent to us. We were so nervous they'd restrict what we could film, but everyone was so generous.

There was an air of giddiness that overtook everyone. It was Daddy's birthday that week too, so everything felt like a celebration, especially when donations started flooding in. Everything was moving forward. This was going to happen. *The Ray D'Arcy Show* invited Colin into the studio and he got filmed there, and the Shanes filmed more scenes at the house. All I had to do was sit in bed and chat. That was the easy bit.

Colin took me out in the new chair and we ran down the road. I could feel the difference in the new wheelchair straight away. It was really comfortable, especially once it was fully adapted for me. George was at the end shouting, 'Go as fast as you can!' So we did. My dress flew up and I could not stop laughing. Madness – but pure joy.

People even stopped to watch. Marty from the Irish Wheelchair Association checked in with me afterwards and took the chair away for further adjustments. As soon as we got it back, Colin took me down to practice the route. They'd padded out the arms, which weren't straight like regular wheelchair arms – they're angled diagonally instead. They'd padded all the sides with this piping foam stuff and adapted the legs too. Basically, anywhere it had looked or felt like I could move or slip, they'd padded.

It ended up being the best decision. Colin and I went through the whole four kilometres, smooth like butter. On the actual day, though, that route looked so different.

The day before the marathon, we went to the Shelbourne. We were going to stay there for two nights and have a last supper – or in my case, soup and prosecco.

We didn't stay up too late, but it was special. After we arrived back at my room, there was a massive bouquet of flowers waiting. I assumed they were in every room.

'They're not in my room,' George said, checking.

'Is there a card?' one of the crew said.

We spotted a card stuffed in among the flowers. It said, 'We're going to have the best day. I love you. Can't wait to see you. Love, Colin.'

I was floored.

'How can I get these home?' I said. 'I want to keep them.' But I didn't care how – I would manage. It was so cool of Colin to send them. They lasted *ages* too.

On the day of the marathon, we all – me, Mom, Daddy, Catherine, her boyfriend Tiernan, George – waited in a house in Nutley Lane on the marathon route. A lovely family had offered us the use of it and we really needed it because it was chaos. Members of Debra, came down: Alé and Cheryl; Kim was there too.

Then, before I knew it, the marathon was on and I was waiting for Colin to come around the bend. He had run thirty-eight kilometres by the time he got to me. I was so excited to see him finally come along and take the handles of my chair.

'Let's take this baby home,' he said. We were off.

I had a group of support runners. Colin had gardaí around him for his security, but I had my own little unit too – people who knew me, knew my condition and knew what to do if something went wrong. And on the day of the marathon, the bumps – those rough jolts on the road – I barely felt them.

I had warned everyone beforehand, 'If anything happens, just let Catherine deal with it.' My sister, listens to me really well. She and Tiernan flanked me the whole way. Catherine knew exactly what to do if I fell. Tiernan knew how to lift me safely. There were also two medical staff running alongside us, but I knew Catherine would step up if needed and take charge.

I am so proud of my sister. I love her and I am always in awe of the things she achieves, she is an incredible woman. I don't know what I would do without her. I remember years ago she was away on a J-1 one summer and a tragic accident happened in the city where she was staying. A group of young Irish people were out on a balcony when it collapsed. It was terrible. We were so panicked trying to reach Catherine, imagining over and over that it had been her group and her friends. Thankfully, she eventually rang us, and when we heard her voice, alive and crying down the phone, shaken to the core, we were so grateful to be the lucky ones. It sat so heavy on us all in Ireland, I think. When she came back at the end of the summer, I was so glad to be able to hug my sister tight, knowing there were families who couldn't.

I was delighted for Catherine when she met Tiernan. They have been together for over four years now; from the start, they just clicked. Catherine never thought she'd find a man tall enough for her. Then Tiernan walked into her life, well over six foot, and that was that. She told me not long after meeting him that she was in love – I was the second person she told, after him.

Tiernan's not just lovely, he's also dependable. I remember telling him that morning, 'You're my strength today.' And he was.

But the man of the moment was Colin. He was amazing, but about the dangers of the whole exercise – look he wasn't wrong. It hurt like hell after. But the way I saw it? I could do the same damage as was done that day going for a coffee. That's EB. The ground is the same everywhere. If I was going to be in pain, I might as well have something to show for it. And that day, we had planned every step.

The Irish Wheelchair Association had advised me to keep my elbows in, but there were so many people waving at me, how could I? I had to go elbows-out so I could wave to all the people cheering. Colin was pushing away, and that's not easy when you've just run nearly forty kilometres. Even with the best chair it was tough on *both* of us. The gardaí running alongside us were checking in on me constantly, as were Catherine and Tiernan. I remember catching one of the medical crew glancing at Catherine with that look – is she okay? – because of how far I was leaning at times.

We did it, Colin and I. The full marathon as a team. I joined him for the final four kilometres – one for each decade I've survived. And those kilometres were long, probably about a half an hour of Colin running along pushing me. But it flew by. I had four pain relief tablets with me and didn't take a single one. The adrenaline, the atmosphere, the people – it was incredible.

As soon as I finished, they backed an ambulance into a tent so no one would see me being taken out. When I saw that I thought they were going to throw me on a trolley, and I was like, *Absolutely not.* But they said they'd transfer me in the chair itself, and once I saw that it wasn't some big dramatic ordeal, I agreed.

I was wheeled up the ramp into the ambulance and someone – I still don't know who, but they obviously know me well – handed me a glass of prosecco. I was stunned. Prosecco in an ambulance! It was like something from a movie.

Jim Aughney arrived then with a medal for Colin and he put it around his neck. Then Colin took it off, walked over to me and placed it gently around my neck. It was such a lovely moment.

Colin sat with me, him drinking a bottle of water as I held onto my glass of bubbly, sitting there in the ambulance, while the crowds buzzed outside. It was surreal. Then Colin got out and Mom and George got in. I didn't drink the prosecco because I was chatting so much.

Dad, Tiernan, Catherine and Colin walked to the Shelbourne, while those of us still in the ambulance drove the few metres from the finish line. When we arrived, there were crowds of people cheering and so many faces I knew. I was passed another glass of prosecco. I didn't drink that one either, because by then I was in a lot of pain. And it wasn't with EB.

I'll tell this next story because I want to make everyone else laugh, but, believe me, I was not laughing at the time.

When we got back to the hotel I was given the prosecco and Colin had a glass of Guinness 0.0 handed to him so we could toast the whole thing. We clinked our glasses, but I didn't even take a sip. Not like me, I know! But you see, I don't think I had taken a proper breath yet. The whole thing had been so exciting, and I had been using my full energy just to take it in. My adrenaline was flowing and I was high on life, but I'd been holding my breath a lot of the time, anticipating bumps or turns that might hurt. And that hadn't exactly agreed with me. About five minutes after we crossed the finish line, I got a really bad cramp.

I don't eat and so, at first, I didn't identify that pain as trapped wind, not at all. I didn't know what was wrong at all, I just wished it would right itself.

However, I kept it to myself as always – remember I hate a fuss. They'd only bring me home and I wanted to see everyone and have the craic. I'd power through.

I was in my electric wheelchair. Colin kept looking over, and at one point he said, 'Are you okay?'

I knew if I said anything he would tell me to get out of there. But I didn't want to. I wanted to be part of the celebration for such an amazing achievement.

Of course, George noticed. She reads me like a book. That

eyesight language we have, she was reading mine whether I wanted her to or not.

'I'm grand,' I said.

'You're not grand,' she said, 'what's wrong with you?'

'Ah no,' I insisted, 'I'm grand.'

I must have been grimacing a bit, because Kim looked straight at me and said, 'Emma. What is the matter?'

'I've a bit of pain in my tummy,' I said. She would have got it out of me eventually.

She immediately went to one of the staff and asked if there was somewhere quiet we could go for a minute. The staff member was only too pleased to show us into a side room, but – oh my God – he started chatting to us and would not leave. Eventually George had to say, 'Sorry, we just need to attend to Emma.'

Once he was gone, I admitted it.

'I've a terrible pain,' I said.

'Where is it?' George said.

I rubbed the area.

'Is it like a stitch?' Kim said.

I nodded.

'Emma,' Kim said, and she didn't even lower her voice when she said the next line with all the nonchalance of a mother of small boys, 'I think you need to fart.'

I could not stop laughing.

'I'm not doing that in this room!'

'Right,' said George, 'up you get.'

'I'm not going to fart,' I said.

'You will so,' George said, and she put her arms around me and I put my arms around her and she lifted me up to standing, sort of. Then she leaned back and – the only way to describe it is – she stretched me.

Kim, with a couple of glasses of champagne in her, started to sing a song about farts. Mothers of boys are always quick with the toilet humour.

'Kim,' I said, 'stop! It's worse if I'm laughing.'

But she didn't stop.

I just thought, *This is peak glamour. Colin Farrell is in the next room and here I am clutching my stomach in a room full of old paintings with Kim doing a fart dance in front of me.*

Then, I burped.

I think they were actually disappointed with that.

But once the bubbles escaped on that end, things shifted and they got the fart they wanted. Kim danced around the room, singing about me and farting and all the bubbles.

'Emma did a fart,' she sang, 'Emma did a faaarrt.'

'Must you?' I said, but I was laughing. It was silly and funny.

Before long I was feeling much better. Well as much as any woman could be with her pride on the floor and her best friends dancing around her, both now singing the fart song.

But look, I was delighted. Delighted that I was still here, delighted to be forty, delighted to have a body that still worked. Delighted to share this amazing and special day with so many of my friends.

It's moments like that, when I feel truly *alive*. Like I've been scooped up and dropped right into the middle of real life – not watching from the sidelines but being watched from the sidelines as I fly down Dublin streets in a borrowed wheelchair with people I love running along beside me. It's those moments when I am being laughed with and laughed at by people who care about me. When I am danced with, and when I am *loved*. When I am treated like the woman I am inside and not like the condition I wear on the outside – that's when I thrive.

Those moments when suddenly one friend or another, usually with a few drinks in them, cannot resist commandeering my wheelchair. One time, at a festival, the CEO of Debra, Jimmy, took over, leaving George in the dust. And I mean he took over *running*. Not on smooth tarmac either. He ran down uneven, cobbled footpaths with me half laughing, half begging him to stop.

'Please, Jimmy, PLEASE!' My laughter was not convincing him I was serious.

So he just laughed and hooted and kept going. It was like he was aiming *for* potholes, not away from them.

'Jimmy, you are banned from pushing me ever again,' I said.

Ah sure, he didn't listen. He has done it again since. And I love every minute.

That's the thing about these people – they're *my* people. Look, we let each other down, we make mistakes, we have all hurt each other without knowing it, of that I am certain. But we all show up when it matters and I wouldn't have it any other way.

The night of the marathon, I really saw what an uplift it had brought to the city. I wanted to stay at the party, but it was too much. Everyone wanted photos and I was trying to smile through the pain of EB. George and Kim staged an intervention and got my mom.

'I'm fine,' I told her.

'Emma, we need to do bandages,' she said.

'I want to be down here,' I said. Because I did. I was part of this wonderful thing; Colin and I had made this magic. I wanted to be in the midst of it. EB could not tell me what to do tonight.

Mom went and got Colin.

'Game over, Em,' he told me straight, 'you're done.' He turned to the crew and told them it was done.

'Emma,' he said, 'it's time to go, admit it, this is it, just go and rest and come back down later if you can.'

I shook my head.

'Emma …' Kim just said my name once, like that, and I knew. I had to go.

So I did.

Once Mom got me upstairs, we realised the extent of the damage. My back, thighs, bum, all were really bad. Mom and George changed the bandages there. During the following bandage change we would realise that the jog had caused the denim jeans I had on to scuff against my knees as well as my thighs.

The pain was so bad I couldn't hack it. 'You need to go to bed,' George said, 'you need to lie down.'

'I don't want to,' I said, 'I want to go back down.'

'Have a rest,' my mom said, 'and then go back down.'

I put my head down on the pillow and rested. Then George came in and woke me and told me there were still a few people downstairs if I was up to it.

So we went back down. The party was over by then and most of the people were gone. It was just me, George, Kim, Cheryl and Susan from Debra, and Catherine, Tiernan and Mom. We had a few drinks, but I was still in pain.

At around eleven, I left them all again, went back to the room and cried my eyes out into my pillow. Not from the pain, not really, but from the disappointment.

That is the reality of EB. We had everything planned. The best equipment. The best prep. But EB doesn't care. EB is always in charge. It's like a shadow, following me around, waiting for a moment to strike. Sometimes I imagine it as a person, waiting around the corner to hurt me. Other times it's like I'm on a spinning board and I'm dizzy with it. Some days EB is quiet. Most days, it throws knives.

That night, George stayed in the adjoining room to me. 'Jesus, Emma,' she said, 'you must be in agony.'

I was.

We left the door open between us. Later, when I was in bed, I called out to her and said, 'George, let's just have one last prosecco, just the two of us to end the night on a perfect high.'

So we did. Me in bed in my pyjamas, George in her dressing gown. It was quiet, it was this calm moment, and it was ours.

That's how I ended the night of the marathon: not on stage, not in photos, but in a soft-lit room with my best friend of eleven years, sharing a final glass of prosecco in the dark.

***

I know that my marathon with Colin was really something special. We raised a million euro. Someone in town said I'd 'lifted the whole country'.

Mom listens to RTÉ all the time, so she heard it and told me – Joe Duffy was doing his top ten moments of the year and one of them was me and Colin in the marathon. It went to a public vote and we came in at number one. Joe said, 'When I saw them go past the finish line, I got goosebumps.'

I thought that was the loveliest thing. And, honestly, it felt like that. It was a huge achievement, not just for me but for everyone.

There is always so much encouragement and humanity in getting me over the line.

Epilogue

In reading my book, I hope I've given you the truth about my life: the best times, the worst times and all the times in between. Because that is what memories are, that is what lives are made up of, and mine is no different.

Some of the worst times of my life were the hardest to write, because to write about loss makes you relive it all over again. Those times were sad, but that doesn't mean my life hasn't been wonderful – it really has. The saddest days of my life, having such loss, it means I have really connected and I have really lived.

Writing this book was never a plan, living through it all was more than enough. But somewhere along the line I realised I wanted this life to be captured and written, so future EB patients can read about it and find hope in these stories. And so we started to write, and in the defining stories from forty years, I began to join the dots and everything started connecting in a way I had never noticed before – all the people who show up again and again; all the choices I made and how they laid the building blocks for who I am as a person. I learnt most of all that life is about trust and love, about reaching out and seeing who is reaching back. Every person who turns up for me again and again – at the hospital, on the phone, in a WhatsApp, or at a fundraiser – you're all part of this story too.

My life has been about EB, of course it has, but it has also been about laughing at the worst times and about crying in the best times. It's about music, and asking for help, and going on that roller coaster even though it scares you, even though it might hurt.

I could have stayed in a bubble, I could have spent my life in bed. Maybe it wouldn't have hurt so much. But I knew I had to be the woman I am in my soul; even if she was restricted by this disease, I would find a way to be her, to be Emma.

I don't know what's next, but I know that I get to choose it, and that is something I will never take for granted. Each day that starts with the sun on my face is a good day. Each night that ends with thank yous and goodnights to the people I love is a good night. That's how I see it.

Even now, as I write this from a hospital bed in James's with a full-body infection they can't seem to clear, I'm still grateful. I'm grateful for every head that pops around the door. For every smile that arrives with medication (I'm definitely smiling back for those). For each phone call, each message, every 'How are you?', every voice note and email. I mean that.

I have never wanted people to see me and feel, oh she is so unfortunate. I want you to feel how I feel – I am really fortunate.

One of the things I told my ghostwriter when we started writing this book was that I hoped each reader would really feel the frustration of the lack of inclusivity in Ireland. Yes, we are an ancient country, built piece by piece over the generations. But come on, if there is money for a bike shelter and Dáil bar bills, there must be money to widen a doorway, fix a lift in the train station, or fund basic support for families in need. It's just not good enough that someone can say, 'There's no budget.' Why is there none? Why are you spending it on rubbish? The cost of that bike shelter would have paid for an EB nurse for ten years. And if they took what they spent on one tiny security hut (1.4 million!) they'd pay her for another thirty.

It's not good enough to say there's no budget when we see public money being spent every day. I'm tired of hearing that one department can't help another. If there's leftover money in a Dáil budget, it should go back to the people, not into something unnecessary. Let's be real. A bike shelter is not a priority in a country where disabled people can't get into buildings. Bikes don't need care. People like me do.

To the nurses reading this – I know most of you are incredible. Ninety-nine per cent of the nurses I've met have been kind, gentle and full of heart. But the reason some of the worst moments made it into these pages is because I want people to understand how vulnerable disabled people are in care. We rely completely on others, especially in the moments when we're in agonising pain and someone else is holding the bowl with the pain tablet in it. Please, always remember what it's like to be on the other side, how scary it is to be a patient and how much we need you to listen and to be patient and compassionate.

To businesses, to companies, to everyone in Ireland: please consider supporting Debra. EB is an unimaginably hard condition to live with. There is no easy way through it. But the care, funding and compassion we receive from Debra and its patrons means everything. If you can give even a fiver or a tenner, it makes a difference. We asked the government for funding years ago, and they promised us. They stood in front of us and said we'd get it. But we never did. Watching money go to bike shelters while that promise remains broken – it hurts.

Governments need to stop making false promises to the people who are counting on them. And as long as there are babies being born into this world with EB, or with any disability, we owe it to them to build something better than what came before. We need to make inclusivity a real priority, not something that's last on the list. We need to make sure that using a wheelchair isn't a barrier to freedom, that having a rare condition doesn't mean living in isolation, and that all of us, no matter what body we're in, can share the same streets, schools, buildings, beaches, buses and futures.

I believe in that. I believe in it with everything I have in me.

I'm so happy to be Emma Fogarty. Being Emma has been a blessing. This life has been an incredible journey and I have loved living it. Even during the times when it was hard to exist as me, I still wouldn't change any of it. Not for the world.

I really love you all.

Lots of love,
Emma x

Acknowledgements

I want to thank my mother, my father, my sister and my extended family for being exactly who you are. Everything we've been through has been easier because we've done it together. Whether it's a celebration or a setback, we've always had each other.

To my mother, thank you for standing by me. You're more than a mother. You are the rock I cling to over and over again in the storm. Thank you for being so fearless and steady. There are no words to describe how lucky I feel to have been given to you as a daughter.

To my dad, for always being soft with me. The ying to my mother's yang. You've made things just a little bit easier, giving me that bit of sympathy when I know I have to push through. It means the world. Thank you for working so hard and making sure we had what we needed to be comfortable – we never took that for granted.

To my sister Catherine, it took ten years, but thank God you came along. That's all I can say. You are a wonderful woman. I love everything about you. I love the people you bring into our life. I just love you, Catherine. Full stop.

Thank you to Tiernan for being such a great support.

To my extended family, my aunts, my uncles, my cousins, everything above and more. You've been the best family ever. We may not always run side by side, but our hands are always outstretched to one another. Across the miles, across the seas, wherever we are. That's extraordinary. I'm blessed to have been born a Fogarty and a Bowen.

To the O'Gorman family, thank you for never letting go, for always coming around my door when I need it, for what you mean to me, and for the patience and love you have shown me my whole life.

To my grandmothers who have passed.

To my friend Bobby, I hope you're looking down from heaven and thinking I've done you proud. I think of you all the time, especially when I'm facing something hard. I don't have you ahead of me any more, but I have you in the place I know I will go to one day. And when I do, I can't wait to see you and tell you all the mad stuff that's been going on since you left. I miss you terribly. Bye for now.

To my friends, Kim, Caitriona and Lynn. For the last laugh we had (which was one of the best) and every laugh before it. For all the laughs still to come. When I think of you, I light up inside. When I hear you coming, I know I'm about to have a great time. I love you guys. I love your partners and your children like they're my own. You're my squad. You've brought joy, humour and steadiness when I've needed it most.

To Pauline and Judith, your care and loyalty has always meant the world to me.

To my PAs, Georgina and Natasha. You help me live. You help me move. You help me make things happen. You give me the independence I crave.

Georgina, what can I say? When I'm an old woman, I hope you're beside me, both of us holding a glass of bubbly. You always turn up for me. You always put me first. You fulfil your role with grace, kindness and strength. You advocate for me, stand up for me, laugh with me. We joke that it's a PA-ship, but this is a real friendship. When I'm old and someone asks me about my friends, your name will be up there.

To Colin Farrell, aka my Col, thank you for writing the foreword, for reading every word, and for understanding the spirit of this story. You're a great pal. I'll never forget the night you sat beside me at dinner. I knew then you had my back, and I'll never stop being grateful for that. Thanks for always being exactly yourself, and for understanding me in the way that you do. You're the best.

To Kathy, Bernadette, Clyde and Abigail, thank you for being just a call or a message away. You're lifelines. You've brought me experiences I'd never have had if I hadn't met you. Clyde, thank you for the fun, for inviting me to your wedding and for giving me that wild boat story. It's a brilliant one at dinner parties.

To Sarah and Aoife, my Christmas visitors, thank you for always showing up for me, in every sense. I'll never forget your kindness during my hardest days, and I hope that on yours I have showed up in the same way.

Thank you to Trisha, for always believing in me. Not just supporting me online, but supporting me personally, in ways that truly mattered. For the 40km you walked on the Camino, thinking and praying for me all the way, even though you didn't know how unwell I really was. That means more than I can say.

To the Debra Ireland community, the board, especially Michael and Jimmy, our CEO. To the OGs: Kim, Susan, Cheryl and Deirdre, thank you for your years of heart and hard work. To the newer members of the team, thank you for showing up with such energy and care. I'm proud to pass the torch to you. Though, if I'm honest, I'm not quite ready to let it go.

To the EB community, thank you for being my mirror.

Thank you for knowing what this life is. For your bravery, your brilliance. We are a community bound by our skin, and we will always be there for each other.

To all of the nurses and doctors who've made life with EB possible: Mary and Denise, my primary public health nurses; Sheila, Catriona and Anne from Bayada; Eimear and Holly at St James's; Mr Ormonde and Dr Gale. And a really special thank you to Dr Rosemarie Watson. You've cared for me since I was a baby. Your work is invisible to most, but I carry it with me every single day. I am so lucky you became a doctor.

To Johnny Sexton, Ray D'Arcy and all the patrons who have supported Debra over the years, especially Perry and Sandy. Thank you for your consistency, your visibility and your humanity. You've used your platform to change lives.

To Killashee House – where do I begin? For the warmth and kindness, for that spot by the window, for the garden, the smiles, the little touches of care, thank you. To Ger Alley, to Orla McCabe, to Paul, Isabella and Zara and all the Kilashee staff who never fail to make us feel at home: your hospitality means the world. For the proseccos, the chocolate swirls and the never-ending welcomes – I appreciate it all, more than I can say.

To everyone at Merrion Press – Conor Graham, my editor Wendy, and to Síne and Ciara – thank you for encouraging me to write this. And to Liosa Mac, thank you for writing this book with me. I've loved every second of it.

To Taylor Swift, your music is not just the soundtrack to my life. It's the spirit of everything I have lived with and lived through. Thank you for being so brave and for sharing your talent with us. You give me an escape when I need it most. You give me somewhere far away to go. Thank you for letting us use your music for the documentary. I still can't believe you watched three minutes of my life and decided to back it. You really are the best and I wish you all the love and happiness in the world.

To Ed Sheeran, your songs have been with me on my darkest days and best nights. Thank you for the music, the comfort and for just being you.

To all the friends and supporters I have met along the way, there are too many of you to mention by name, but thank you so much for everything, all the times you have stepped forward, all the times you have given something – time, money, a helping hand, even just sharing a story or reposting something – thank you!

And finally, to everyone reading this: if you've ever felt invisible, pushed aside, or like you've had to fight for space in your own story, I hope this book proves that your story matters. It can be told. It can be heard. And maybe, just maybe, it will be felt by someone else and will give them hope too.

Let's pass that light back and forth.

Carpe diem, seize the day.